YOGA FOR HEALTH

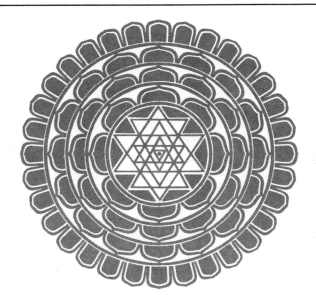

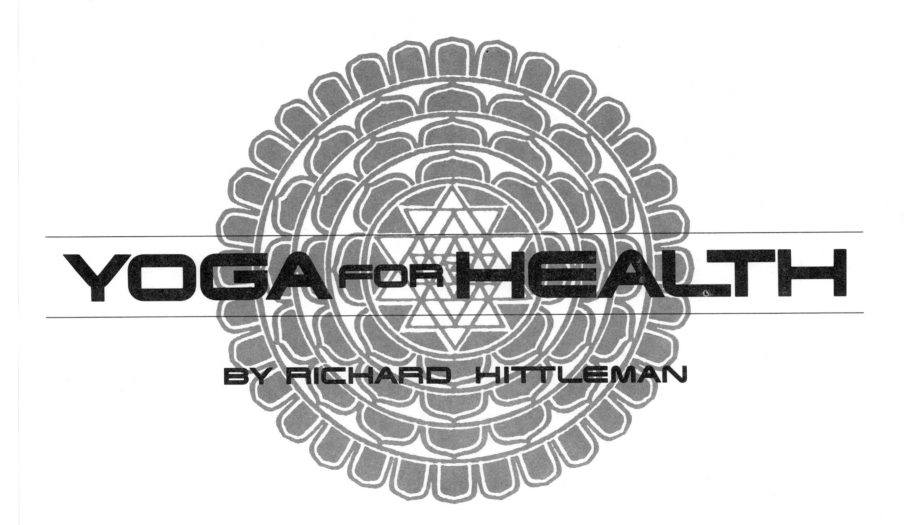

YOGA FOR HEALTH

BY RICHARD HITTLEMAN

BALLANTINE BOOKS • NEW YORK

Library of Congress Catalog Card Number: 82-90825
ISBN: 0-345-32798-5

Photographs: Thomas Burke
Models: Lisa Moody and Greg Hittleman
Design by Michaelis/Carpelis Design Associates, Inc.

Manufactured in the United States of America

First Edition: April 1983

14 15 16 17 18 19 20

To those great Yogis, whose compassion moved them to reveal
the means by which physical, mental, and emotional sufferings
may be terminated, this book is respectfully dedicated.

PREFACE

This book contains the basic materials of the Yoga for Health System which I have developed during twenty-five years of teaching and which has enabled several million people in the western world to experience numerous benefits inherent in the Yoga science.

The emphasis of the system is on simplicity and practicality; it renders the Yoga principles immediately applicable by people of all ages and with many different physical and philosophical backgrounds. Minimal preparation is necessary. You can begin your use of the materials in all four sections of this book today.

Being thoroughly familiar with the effectiveness of the Yoga For Health system, I can tell you without reservation that those who devote their efforts to its application are never disappointed. Perform a daily routine of *Hatha Yoga*; apply the nutrition principles; try the food recipes; reflect upon the philosophy; experiment with the meditation techniques. You will soon attain a level of health and serenity that you could not have previously imagined.

Always be aware that the permanent fulfillment you are seeking lies within. Gradually you will recognize Yoga—even in its physical context—as that profound practice which turns you inward and guides you, gently but unswervingly, along the inner path.

Health and Peace,

Richard J. Hittleman
Yoga Universal

Richard Hittleman

CONTENTS

PART I HATHA YOGA

Introduction _____ 3
  1. Chest Expansion _____ 6
  2. Triangle _____ 8
  3. Rishi's Posture _____ 10
  4. Balance Posture _____ 12
  5. Roll Twist _____ 14
  6. Dancer's Posture _____ 16
  7. Knee and Thigh Stretch _____ 18
  8. Twist _____ 20
  9. Back Stretch _____ 22
 10. Alternate Leg Stretch _____ 24
 11. Backward Bend _____ 26
 12. Cobra _____ 28
 13. Neck Movements _____ 30
 14. Locust _____ 32
 15. Bow _____ 34
 16. Side Raise _____ 36
 17. Back Push Up _____ 38
 18. Shoulder Stand _____ 40
 19. Plough _____ 44
 20. Complete Breath _____ 46
Three Advanced Exercises _____
 21. Abdominal Lift _____ 48
 22. Head Stand _____ 50
 23. Lotus Postures _____ 54

24. Special Routine _____ 58
Relaxation-Meditation Techniques _____
25. Deep Relaxation _____ 62
26. Alternate Nostril Breathing _____ 64
27. Directing the Life Force _____ 66
Practice Plan _____ 68
Yoga for Problems _____ 70

PART II NUTRITION

Introduction _____ 75
Food Classification _____ 78
   Fruits _____ 78
   Vegetables _____ 79
   Proteins _____ 81
   Dairy Products _____ 85
   Seasonings _____ 87
   Sugar _____ 88
   Beverages _____ 89
   Food Supplements _____ 91
   Summary Charts _____ 92
Menus _____ 94
   Lunch Box Suggestions _____ 98
Sources of the Recommended Foods _____ 98
Weight Regulation _____ 99
Family, Social, and Restaurant Dining _____ 101
Fasting _____ 102

PART III RECIPES

   Notes _____ 106
   Suggested Appliances and Utensils _____ 107
   Homemade Yogurt _____ 107
Appetizers, Spreads _____ 108
Beverages _____ 112

Soups _____ 116
Salads _____ 122
Dressings _____ 129
Main Dishes _____ 132
Breads and Muffins _____ 148
Cereals _____ 150
Waffles, Pancakes _____ 152
Fruit Desserts _____ 153
Puddings and Custards _____ 157
Ice Cream and Sherbet _____ 159
Pastries _____ 160
Candies and Other Sweet Treats _____ 165

PART IV PHILOSOPHY AND MEDITATION

Principles _____ 168
  1. What We are Not _____ 168
  2. The World Within the Mind _____ 172
  3. Reincarnation: The Consequence of Desire _____ 177
  4. The Illusion of "Identity" _____ 180
  5. Action Without *Karma* _____ 184
  6. The False God of the Ego _____ 185
  7. Function of the Guru _____ 189
  8. Yoga, the Universal Practice for Here and Now _____ 192
Meditation _____ 194
  Observation of the Breath _____ 196
  Yantra _____ 196
  OM _____ 198
  Candle _____ 199
  Alternate Nostril Breathing _____ 200
  Flower _____ 201
  Incense _____ 202
  Touch _____ 204
  Surrender of the Ego _____ 205
  Where Am I? _____ 206

PART I
HATHA YOGA

INTRODUCTION

This section contains exercises that are known in Sanskrit as *asanas,* meaning postures or poses. The total series of *asanas* is designated as *Hatha* (physical) Yoga. A select, highly effective group of these comprises the basic exercise program of the Yoga For Health system. This program is presented in the following pages.

In undertaking the practice of *Hatha* Yoga, you are joining millions of people throughout the world who have turned to this most ancient and respected of natural methods for achieving and maintaining a high level of physical, mental, and emotional health. These people, of all ages and backgrounds, have found Yoga to be the perfect lifetime fitness program.

You will probably be pleasantly surprised, if not actually astonished, at how easy most of the movements are and how quickly you experience positive results. You can begin the Yoga practice nearly regardless of your age or present physical condition.

This is because you are not in competition with anyone; you do only what *you* can do comfortably, at your own pace, without strain, without huffing and puffing, without feeling you have benefited only when you are on the verge of collapse, as is the case in many systems of exercise. Beginning students frequently say, "I don't know if I can do these exercises." My response is, "If you can move your body one inch in any direction, you can do sufficient Yoga to experience significant benefits almost at once." This is true because while the movements can be performed in as simple a manner as is comfortable for you, they are extremely profound in nature. They reach deep into the organism; they massage, stimulate, relieve tension, work out stiffness, release trapped energy, revitalize, and assist in overcoming many physical and emotional problems. Whereas most methods of physical conditioning emphasize the muscular system, Yoga addresses *all* systems of the body: muscular,

endocrine, respiratory, nervous, etc.

The approach to Yoga practice is totally different from that of calisthenics. First, you quiet the mind and emotions. Then, performing the exercises, you move for the most part slowly, with the poise, rhythm, and concentration of a dancer. You perform few repetitions of each exercise; postures such as the Shoulder and Head Stands are done only once during a practice session. You hold your extreme position for a brief interval while your mind is fully focused on what the body is feeling. You sink into the movements, you become the movements, you have a joyous physical experience in knowing and understanding your body from a new perspective. Indeed, *Hatha* Yoga assists you in perceiving the spiritual reality of your existence and, as stated by the ancient gurus, "is that practice which renders the mind fit for meditation." So it is essential to be aware that when you are engaged in *Hatha* Yoga there is much more involved than physical movement and exercising. You will soon come to understand the truth of this, and you will look forward to your practice session as one of the most enjoyable and meaningful periods of the day.

During the next several weeks, devote as much time as you can each day to learning the positions. Begin with the first *asana,* and work your way through to the end of the section. Then repeat the procedure a number of times until you feel you understand what is involved with each *asana.* Be certain to follow all of the instructions for performing, holding, and repeating exactly as written. *Never strain;* never go further than is comfortable. There is no hurry to attain an extreme position. The beginning and intermediate positions hold as much benefit for you while you are learning as the extreme positions will later on. If you hurry or strain, you will retard your progress. Learning the positions in this methodical, progressive manner will impart a sense of satisfaction, and you will continue to derive the various benefits listed below. Do not skip any of the postures. If any seems particularly difficult, do whatever modified position you can. A bend, stretch, lift, or inversion of only a few inches will prove beneficial.

Here is what you need to consider in preparing to practice: Allow at least ninety minutes to elapse after eating. Attempt to practice at the same hour each day. Minimal clothing is desirable; you must have complete freedom of movement, so nothing tight or restrictive should be worn. Remove watch, eyeglasses, and jewelry. Locate a flat surface with sufficient space for you to stretch in all directions. Select an area that is private and where you will not be disturbed. Cover this flat surface with a thin mat or large towel five to six feet long and approximately three feet wide. Use this covering only for your practice. Ideally, your practice environment (indoors or outdoors) should be conducive to a serene, elevating mode of mind, and there should be a supply of fresh air. However, these conditions are frequently difficult to meet and are not essential. The main factor is that wherever you practice, you do so patiently, seriously, and regularly. You will want to time yourself in various "holding" positions, so place a silent clock or watch where the seconds and minutes can be easily read. The Locust and Head Stand postures may be facilitated by the use of a small pillow approximately six inches in height. Place this in the practice area before you begin. Once begun, practice should never be interrupted by your needing to obtain articles or by any activity that requires you to leave the area.

There will be days during which your body may not respond as well as it did the day before. Students frequently evaluate this as a "setback" and become discouraged. However, this is not a real regression. The body is simply pulling back a little in order to set itself firmly into the positions you have been teaching it. If you are patient on these days and go through your practice session to the best of your ability, you will assist the body in setting, and in a day or two it will be ready to move ahead once again. Permitting the body to set itself in this manner will enable you to derive benefits at each step of the way, and you will make steady progress. The body will learn the positions so thoroughly that it will never forget them, and you will be able to execute all of the postures throughout your entire life. I know from my personal experience with thousands of class students that the flexibility and other youthful physical characteristics developed through serious Yoga practice are maintained for life.

Once you have become familiar with the *asanas* through this learning procedure, your practice should take the form indicated in the Practice Plan at the end of this section. By faithfully following this plan with thirty to forty minutes of daily practice sessions, and adopting the principles contained in the other sections of this book, you can expect to:

• Develop strength and muscle tone in all areas of the body.
• Increase endurance and heighten resistance to many common disorders.
• Maintain lifelong flexibility in spine and limbs.
• Eliminate tension, and quiet the mind and emotions as necessary.
• Release trapped energies and gain access to untapped Life-Force.
• Improve efficiency in all activities through steadiness of mind.
• Acquire greater control of the body through cultivation of balance and poise.
• Overcome various negative conditions of the body such as stiffness, congestion, nervousness.
• Promote the regulation and redistribution of weight.

If you are currently involved in jogging, the martial arts, golf, etc., and you believe these things to be of genuine value, you can continue to engage in them. However, understand that your Yoga practice is a totally different activity and should be undertaken entirely apart from these sports. Most sports *promote* stress and tension; it is interesting to note that many people have found it highly beneficial to loosen and relax themselves with a brief routine of the *asanas* prior to or immediately following a sporting event, as well as prior to a business meeting, school examination, or any activity in which they want to be particularly alert and yet relaxed. It won't take long to discover which of the *asanas* are effective for your particular needs in this regard. However, such application of the *asanas* should not be regarded as actual practice. Serious use of the postures in a therapeutic context is described on pages 70-71.

Read through the Nutrition section as soon as possible, and attempt to incorporate these principles into your diet. The benefits of *Hatha* Yoga practice will be increased through adoption of these principles.

It is suggested that you consult your physician before undertaking any system of exercise. Because of its nonstrenuous nature and involvement with all body systems, an increasing number of medical and health authorities are recommending Yoga practice to their patients.

You now know everything necessary to begin your practice. Devote yourself seriously to *Hatha* Yoga for the next few weeks and you will begin to understand its extraordinary value and why it has endured these many centuries. Regard your practice session as that time which totally transcends your ordinary life. You transport yourself into another dimension of existence where your mind and senses are turned wholly within. It is in this dimension that you draw ever closer to the source of your being. And it is that source which restores your health, replenishes your energies, and maintains your life.

CHEST EXPANSION

BENEFITS

Removes tension throughout spine, neck, and shoulders.

•

Develops, strengthens, and firms chest and bust.

•

Firms upper arms.

•

Improves posture.

•

Refreshes brain with increased blood supply.

•

Helps to increase lung capacity.

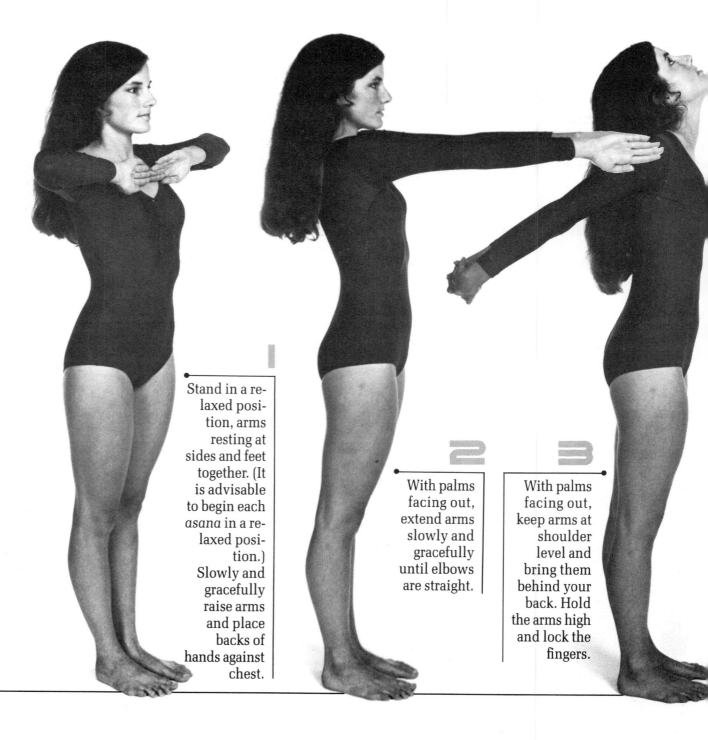

1

• Stand in a relaxed position, arms resting at sides and feet together. (It is advisable to begin each *asana* in a relaxed position.) Slowly and gracefully raise arms and place backs of hands against chest.

2

• With palms facing out, extend arms slowly and gracefully until elbows are straight.

3

• With palms facing out, keep arms at shoulder level and bring them behind your back. Hold the arms high and lock the fingers.

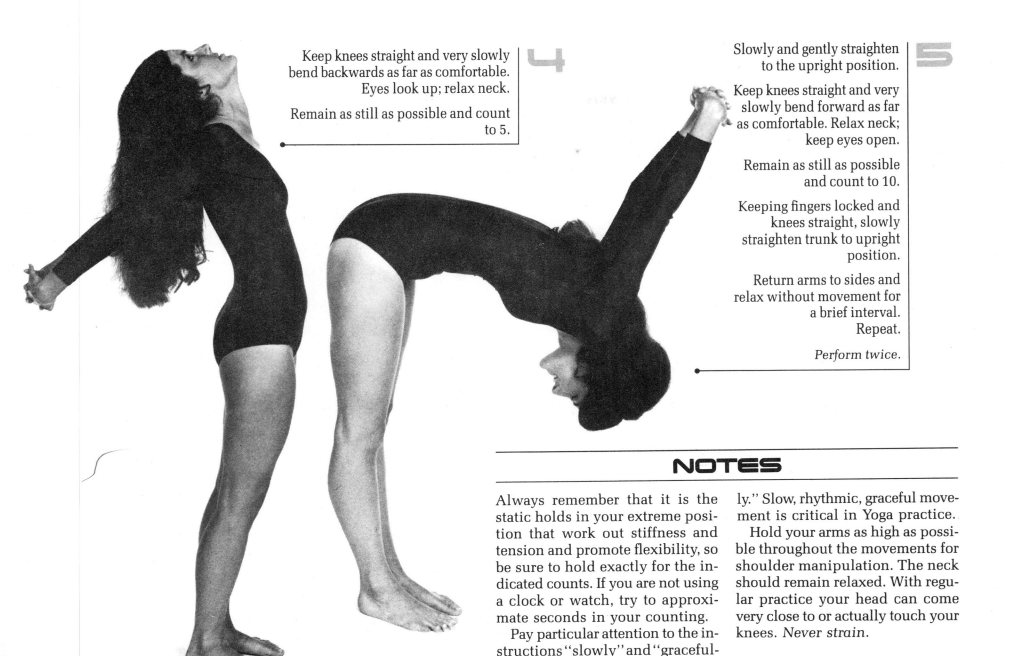

4

Keep knees straight and very slowly bend backwards as far as comfortable. Eyes look up; relax neck.

Remain as still as possible and count to 5.

5

Slowly and gently straighten to the upright position.

Keep knees straight and very slowly bend forward as far as comfortable. Relax neck; keep eyes open.

Remain as still as possible and count to 10.

Keeping fingers locked and knees straight, slowly straighten trunk to upright position.

Return arms to sides and relax without movement for a brief interval. Repeat.

Perform twice.

NOTES

Always remember that it is the static holds in your extreme position that work out stiffness and tension and promote flexibility, so be sure to hold exactly for the indicated counts. If you are not using a clock or watch, try to approximate seconds in your counting.

Pay particular attention to the instructions "slowly" and "gracefully." Slow, rhythmic, graceful movement is critical in Yoga practice.

Hold your arms as high as possible throughout the movements for shoulder manipulation. The neck should remain relaxed. With regular practice your head can come very close to or actually touch your knees. *Never strain.*

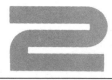

2 TRIANGLE

BENEFITS

Firms the sides.
•
Firms the thighs.
•
Streamlines the waist.
•
A good movement for those with tightness and other problems in the shoulders.

1

Assume a stance with the legs two to three feet apart. Slowly raise arms to shoulder level, with palms facing down.

2

Keeping knees straight and neck relaxed, slowly bend trunk to left, and take a firm hold on the lowermost area that left hand can reach.

As you bend to the left, bring the right arm, with elbow straight, over the head so that it is held approximately parallel to the floor.

Remain frozen in this position while you count to 10.

Very slowly return trunk and arms to the position of Figure 1.

Bend slowly to the right and perform the same movements.

3

You will be able to attain the more extreme positions with practice. In Figure 3 the model has gained sufficient suppleness to reach the ankle.

Very slowly return trunk and arms to position of Figure 1. Repeat.

Following final repetition, slowly bring feet together and simultaneously lower arms to sides. Relax without movement for a brief interval.

Perform three times to each side, alternating left and right.

NOTES

Note that Figure 3 depicts a wider stance than that of Figure 2. As you increase your proficiency in this *asana*, you can widen your stance for a more intensive stretch.

For maximum firming, the arm must be brought over the head with the palm facing down and the elbow straight.

Very slow movement in returning the trunk to the upright position will strengthen and firm the thighs, calves, and waist.

3 RISHI'S POSTURE

BENEFITS

Strengthens the back and spine through intensive twisting movements.

•

Promotes flexibility and poise.

•

Aids in equalizing the sides.

•

Streamlines the waist.

1 In a standing position, slowly raise arms, palms down, to chest level.

2 Keeping the knees straight, slowly bend the trunk forward and slide the right hand down the inside of the right leg.

At the same time, with the elbow straight, bring the left arm behind the back. Eyes follow the back of the left hand as it moves behind you. Continue to bend the trunk forward as far as possible. At this point the right hand takes a firm hold on the side and back of the right leg.

Hold as steady as possible for a count of 10.

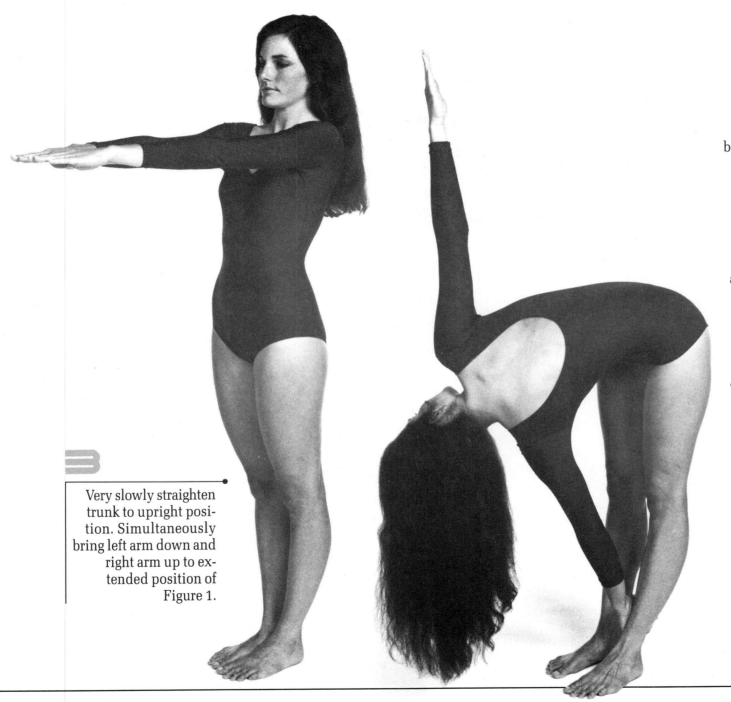

Bend forward slowly, and slide the left hand down the left leg with the right hand moving behind you. Perform the same movements and hold for a count of 10.

Straighten up as described above. Repeat.

Following final repetition, slowly lower arms to sides and relax without movement for a brief interval.

Perform twice on each side, alternating left and right.

4

NOTES

You will often find that one side of the body is more limber than the other. There are several Yoga techniques that help correct this condition; Rishi's Posture is one.

Be sure to hold the leg firmly and perform an intensive twist of the trunk against this hold. If you cannot see the back of the upraised hand, you have raised it too high. Do not bend the knees at any point.

3

Very slowly straighten trunk to upright position. Simultaneously bring left arm down and right arm up to extended position of Figure 1.

4 BALANCE POSTURE

BENEFITS

Promotes excellent balance.
•
Relieves tension in back and shoulders.

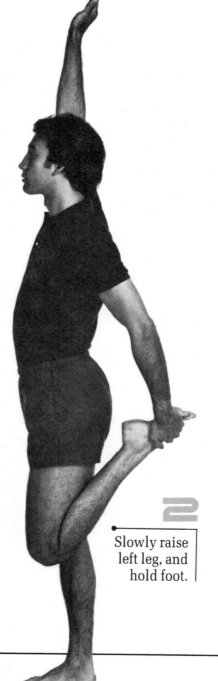

1 With feet together, slowly raise right arm straight upward. Elbow is straight.

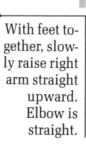

2 Slowly raise left leg, and hold foot.

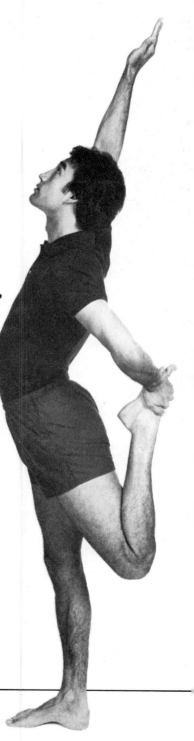

3 Slowly bend trunk and head slightly backward and gently pull left foot upward toward lower back.

Pull very gently; do not strain. Eyes look upward; right elbow remains straight.

Hold as steady as possible for a count of 5.

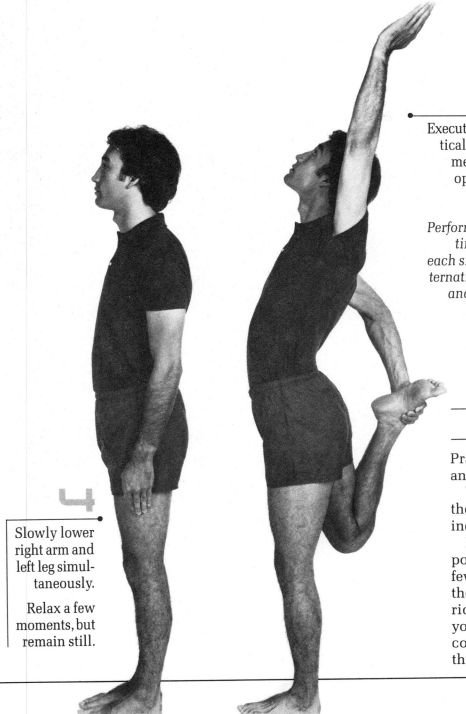

Execute identical movements on opposite side.

Perform three times on each side, alternating left and right.

4

Slowly lower right arm and left leg simultaneously.

Relax a few moments, but remain still.

NOTES

Practice to achieve smoothness and continuity in the movements.

Your balance may be erratic in the beginning, but steadiness will increase with practice.

If you lose your balance at any point during the exercise, pause a few moments and try again from the beginning position. Keep a serious attitude; do not laugh at yourself, and never become discouraged. Success is achieved through persistence.

If, during initial attempts, you find it absolutely impossible to maintain your balance, you may place the side of the upraised arm against a wall. But continue to attempt the exercise without the aid.

Gaining control of your balance enhances all your movements (walking, running, dancing, sports), increases confidence, and imparts a feeling of "lightness" to the entire body.

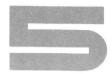

5
ROLL
TWIST

BENEFITS

Reduces excess weight and inches in waist and hips.

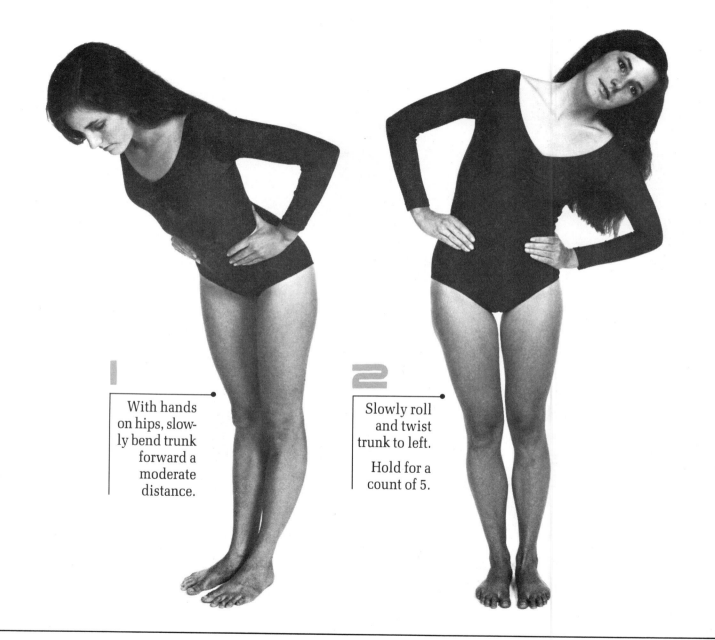

1 With hands on hips, slowly bend trunk forward a moderate distance.

2 Slowly roll and twist trunk to left.

Hold for a count of 5.

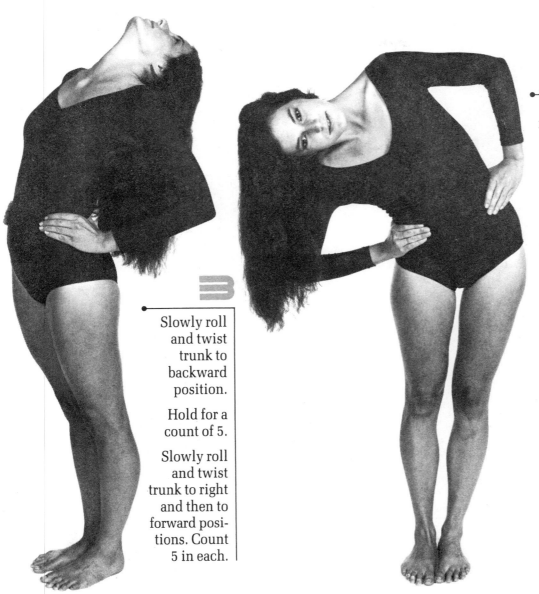

3

Slowly roll and twist trunk to backward position.

Hold for a count of 5.

Slowly roll and twist trunk to right and then to forward positions. Count 5 in each.

4

Execute identical movements in the opposite direction: roll and twist trunk from forward position to right, backward, and left positions. Count 5 in each hold.

Following final repetition, slowly straighten trunk to upright position and return arms to sides. Relax, but remain still for a brief interval.

Perform three times in each direction, alternating directions.

NOTES

Be sure that you do not simply *bend* the trunk into the positions, but that you *roll and twist* with exaggerated movements in the waist and hips.

The illustration depicts a more extreme position. You can attempt this wider circle after several weeks of practice.

Keep in mind that you are attempting to make a perfect circle with your trunk by rolling and twisting the same distance to each position.

6
DANCER'S POSTURE
BENEFITS

Firms and strengthens legs.

Strengthens feet and ankles.

Promotes balance.

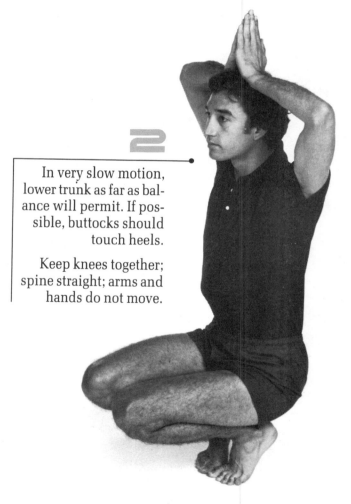

1 With feet together, place palms overhead as illustrated.

2 In very slow motion, lower trunk as far as balance will permit. If possible, buttocks should touch heels.

Keep knees together; spine straight; arms and hands do not move.

3

When trunk has been lowered as far as possible, do not pause but immediately begin to raise trunk, in very slow motion, to upright position, and come up onto toes.

Hold as steady as possible for a count of 5.

Return soles of feet to floor, and repeat.

Following final repetition, slowly return arms to sides. Relax, but remain still for a brief interval.

Perform five times.

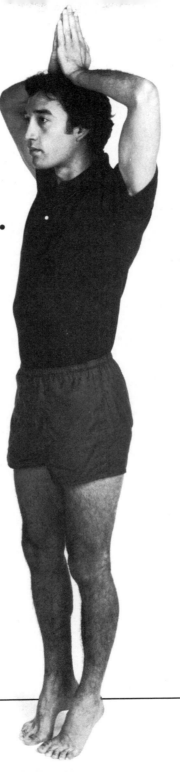

NOTES

Steadiness in balance and the ability to touch buttocks to heels will develop with practice.

Moving as slowly as possible, especially in the upward movement, will greatly strengthen the legs. Holding the position on the toes will strengthen the ankles and feet.

Keeping the knees together optimizes benefits.

If you lose your balance at any point, pause a few moments and begin again.

7
KNEE AND THIGH STRETCH

BENEFITS

Works out tightness and relieves tension in knees and thighs.

•

Strengthens knees.

•

Firms thighs.

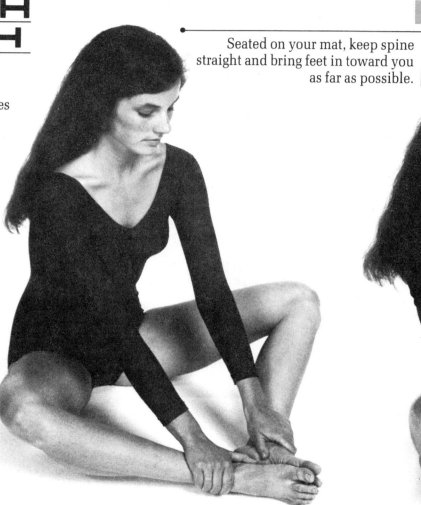

1

Seated on your mat, keep spine straight and bring feet in toward you as far as possible.

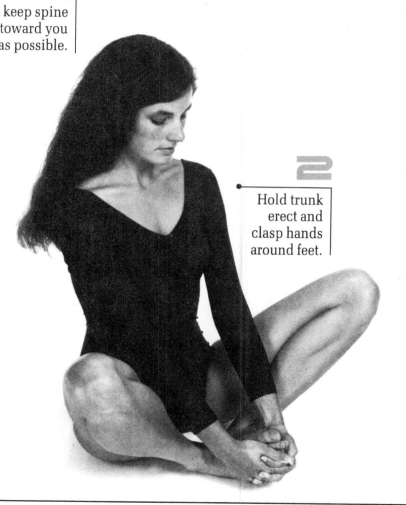

2

Hold trunk erect and clasp hands around feet.

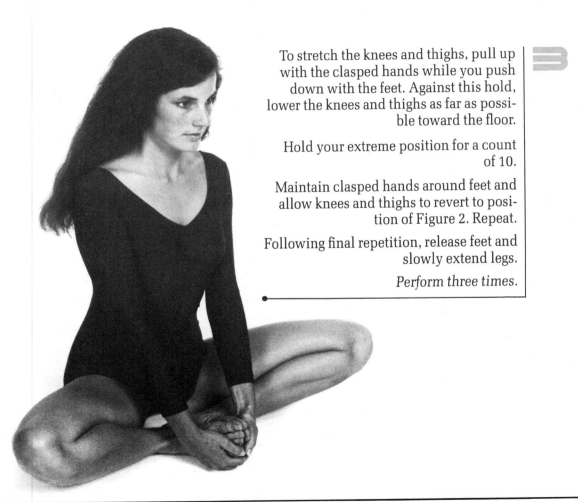

To stretch the knees and thighs, pull up with the clasped hands while you push down with the feet. Against this hold, lower the knees and thighs as far as possible toward the floor.

Hold your extreme position for a count of 10.

Maintain clasped hands around feet and allow knees and thighs to revert to position of Figure 2. Repeat.

Following final repetition, release feet and slowly extend legs.

Perform three times.

NOTES

For many students, the inside upper thigh area is exceptionally tight. This *asana* assists in working out that tightness. Also, the knees are made to bend outward, a healthful movement they seldom make in ordinary activities. Significant tension that accumulates in these areas can be stretched away through this posture.

Figure 3 depicts an extreme stretch, accomplished with practice. In the beginning, lowering the knees even one inch is of value.

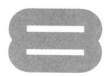

TWIST

BENEFITS

Provides an immediate relief for back and spinal tension.

•

Promotes flexibility.

•

Assists in reducing excess inches in waist.

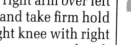

Seated on your mat, extend legs straight outward.

Cross left leg over right and rest sole of left foot on floor. Place left hand on floor behind your back for balance.

Cross right arm *over* left knee and take firm hold of right knee with right hand.

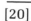

Very slowly turn head and twist trunk as far as possible to the *left*.

Hold for a count of 10. Keep trunk erect.

Slowly return head and trunk to the forward position.

Relax a few moments. Hands remain in the position of Figure 3.

Repeat.

Execute identical movements on opposite side.

Following final repetition, extend both legs straight outward.

Perform three times on left side, then three times on right side.

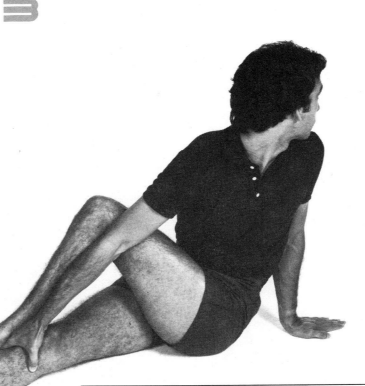

NOTES

At first you may feel cramped in all movements of the exercise. This will disappear with practice.

Be sure that you have assumed the correct position in Figure 2. The arm crosses *over* the opposite knee.

In Figure 3, be sure that you are twisting in the correct direction. Your trunk is held erect, and the head must turn with the trunk to the extreme position. Turning the head and bringing the cervical vertebrae into play makes the twist complete.

The vertebrae respond well to this "corkscrew" movement. Spinal twisting is a standard technique of the chiropractor. Students frequently feel highly exhilarated after this exercise because there is an immediate loosening of the back and spine and a resultant freeing of energy.

9
BACK STRETCH
BENEFITS

Relieves tension throughout the body.

•

Promotes lifelong flexibility.

•

Strengthens back and spine.

•

Stretches and firms legs.

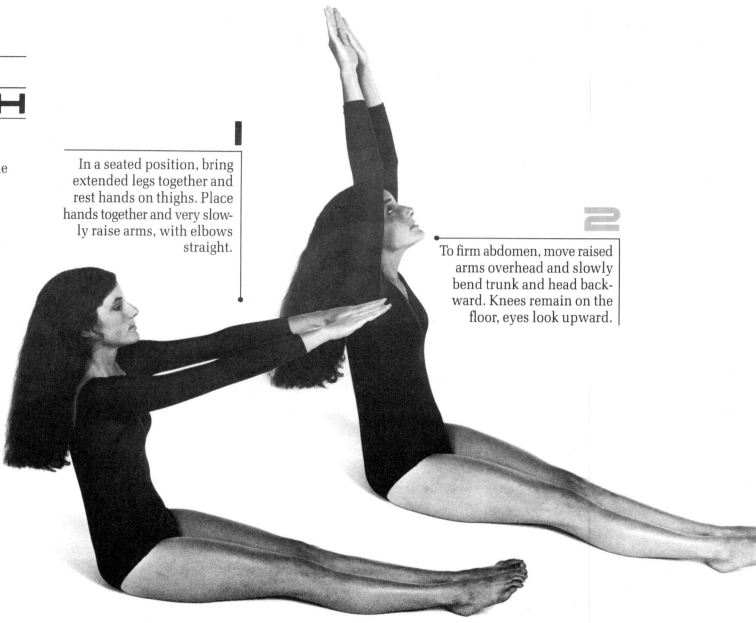

1

In a seated position, bring extended legs together and rest hands on thighs. Place hands together and very slowly raise arms, with elbows straight.

2

To firm abdomen, move raised arms overhead and slowly bend trunk and head backward. Knees remain on the floor, eyes look upward.

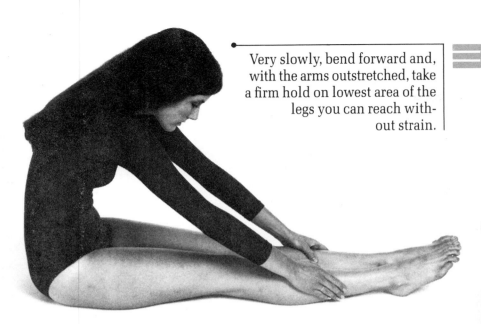

3 Very slowly, bend forward and, with the arms outstretched, take a firm hold on lowest area of the legs you can reach without strain.

4 Against the hold you have on the legs, very slowly lower the trunk as far as possible without strain.

Keep neck relaxed to stretch cervical vertebrae. Backs of knees must remain on floor.

Hold for a count of 10.

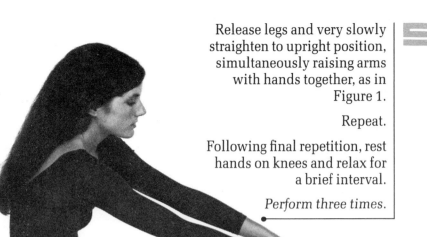

5 Release legs and very slowly straighten to upright position, simultaneously raising arms with hands together, as in Figure 1.

Repeat.

Following final repetition, rest hands on knees and relax for a brief interval.

Perform three times.

NOTES

This is one of the most powerful series of movements through which spinal flexibility and strengthening of the back can be achieved and maintained.

As with the Chest Expansion, this *asana* can be performed at any time of the day when a relief of back tension is indicated.

You will be pleasantly surprised at how quickly an extreme degree of flexibility is developed through the Back Stretch. Very soon you may be able to hold your feet and rest your head on your knees (as shown in Figure 4).

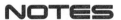

10
ALTERNATE LEG STRETCH

BENEFITS

Removes tension, strengthens and firms the legs.
•
Strengthens and firms each side of the lower back.

2 Slowly raise arms to overhead position; bend trunk backward several inches; look upward.

3 Execute slow dive forward, and firmly hold the furthermost part of left leg that can be reached without strain.

1 Legs are extended. Take right foot with hands and place it so that heel is as far in toward you as possible and sole rests against inside of left thigh.

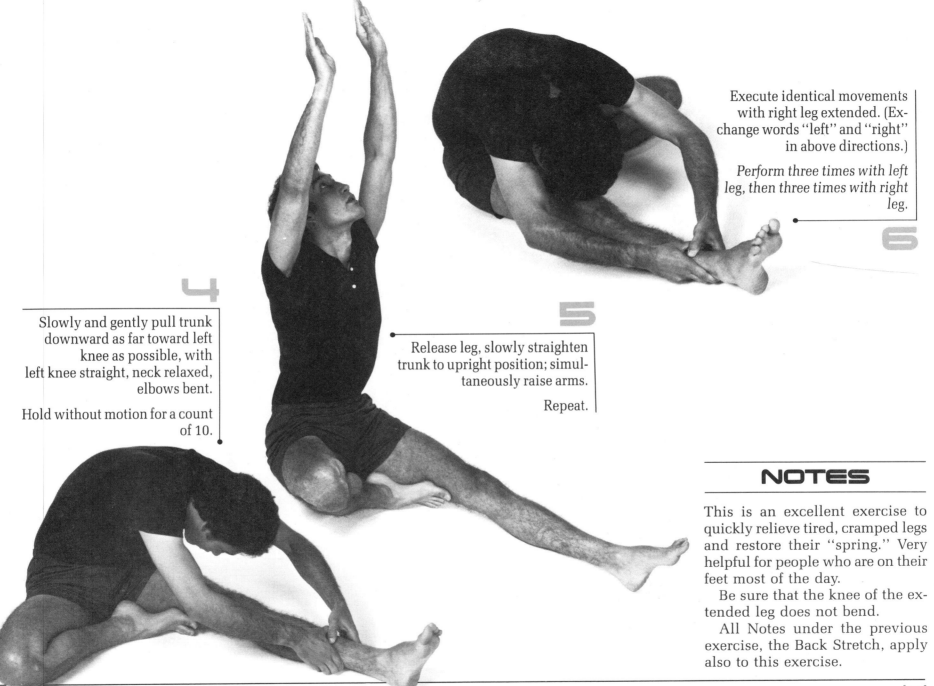

6

Execute identical movements with right leg extended. (Exchange words "left" and "right" in above directions.)

Perform three times with left leg, then three times with right leg.

4

Slowly and gently pull trunk downward as far toward left knee as possible, with left knee straight, neck relaxed, elbows bent.

Hold without motion for a count of 10.

5

Release leg, slowly straighten trunk to upright position; simultaneously raise arms.

Repeat.

NOTES

This is an excellent exercise to quickly relieve tired, cramped legs and restore their "spring." Very helpful for people who are on their feet most of the day.

Be sure that the knee of the extended leg does not bend.

All Notes under the previous exercise, the Back Stretch, apply also to this exercise.

BACKWARD BEND

BENEFITS

Strengthens, imparts flexibility, and helps remove stiffness and cramps from ankles, feet, and toes.

•

Provides an intensive convex stretch for the back.

•

Increases blood supply to head.

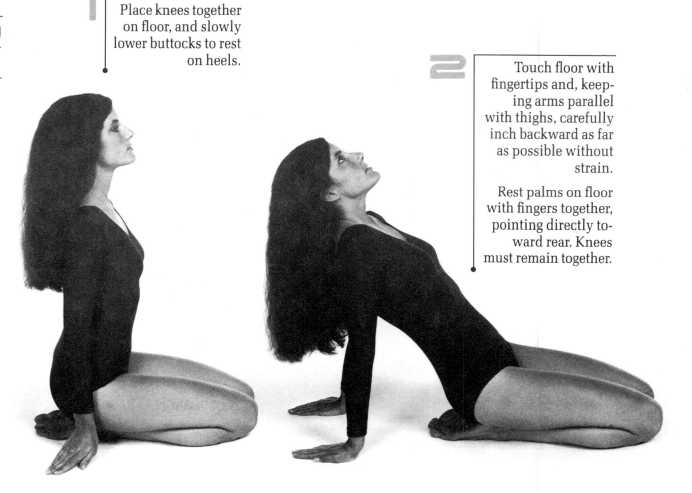

1 Place knees together on floor, and slowly lower buttocks to rest on heels.

2 Touch floor with fingertips and, keeping arms parallel with thighs, carefully inch backward as far as possible without strain.

Rest palms on floor with fingers together, pointing directly toward rear. Knees must remain together.

3

Without raising buttocks from heels, arch the back and bend the head back. Eyes look up.

Hold as steady as possible for a count of 20.

Very slowly, raise head and relax trunk. Inch hands forward to position of Figure 1.

4

Move trunk forward so that toes are in position of Figure 4.

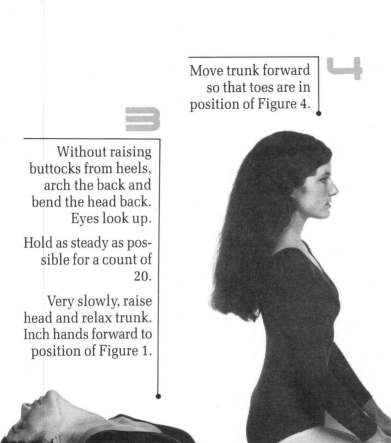

5

Again, touch floor with fingertips and very cautiously perform the same movements. Be sure not to *lunge* backward.

Hold your extreme position for a count of 10.

Very slowly raise head, relax trunk, and inch hands forward to starting position.

Perform each position once. Note that the first position is held for a count of 20 and the second for a count of 10.

NOTES

Be sure that the knees remain together, the arms are parallel with the sides, the fingers are together and point as indicated, the neck is relaxed in the extreme positions, and that the buttocks remain on the heels. Move cautiously and *never* lunge backward or forward.

The Backward Bend positions assist in overcoming stiffness and weakness in the toes, feet, and ankles. The position of Figure 5 is particularly strengthening but must be attained slowly, over a period of time. In the beginning, just sitting on your heels for a few moments at each practice session will gradually enable the feet to support your weight and allow you to add inches to the backward movement.

12
COBRA

BENEFITS

Provides an immediate relief of tension.

Firms and strengthens the arms and lower back.

Promotes flexibility through an intensive convex stretch.

1 Rest forehead on mat. Place hands beneath shoulders; fingers are together and point toward opposite hand.

2 Slowly raise head.

Begin to slowly raise trunk by pushing hands against floor.

3 Continue to very slowly raise trunk. Spine is curved throughout movements.

Reverse movements and very slowly lower trunk to floor. Forehead rests on mat.

Relax entire body for approximately one minute.

Repeat.

Perform twice.

Raise as high as is comfortable.

(In extreme position elbows are straight, head back, lower abdomen touching floor, legs relaxed.)

Hold for a count of 15.

NOTES

There is nothing comparable to the Cobra for relieving tension throughout the back and spine. Each vertebra is stressed and relaxed in turn.

Your head is continually tilted backward. Your spine must be continually arched, never straightened.

Be sure that the hand and finger position is correct: hands beneath shoulders, fingers pointing toward opposite hand.

A slow motion is essential. The slower the movement, the more complete the removal of tension and the greater the strengthening and firming in the back and arms.

Figure 4 depicts the extreme position. But in the beginning, raise your trunk only as high as is comfortable. Your elbows need not be straight, but the spine must be arched, whatever your position. You will probably find yourself raising an inch higher in each practice session.

The Cobra is a technique that has served as highly effective therapy in problems of the back and spine.

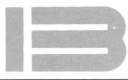

MOVEMENTS
NECK

BENEFITS

Relieves and helps prevent stiffness, tension and cramps in the neck.

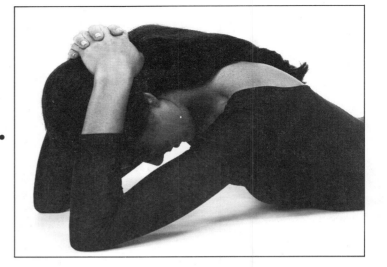

In these movements, the use of the hands enables the head to be lowered and turned farther than would be the case if the hands were not assisting. This extra half-inch of movement is highly effective in getting to the tense areas, so do not rest the head in the hands, but grip it firmly and move it with deliberation.

1. Lie on abdomen and place elbows on floor. Arms are parallel.

2. Use clasped hands to gently push head down so that chin touches chest.

Hold for a count of 10.

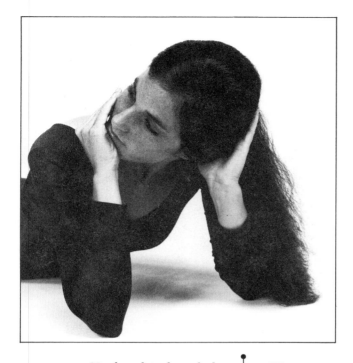

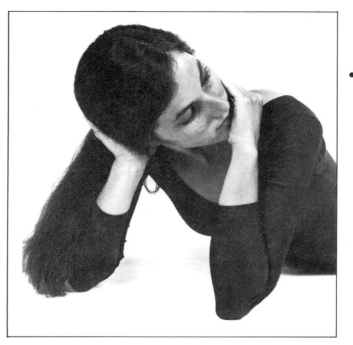

Without moving arms, turn head so that chin rests in right hand. Back of head is firmly held by left hand.

Use hands to slowly and firmly turn head as far as possible to right. Hold extreme position for a count of 10.

Turn head to front position. Repeat.

Following final repetition, lower chin to mat and return arms to sides (in preparation for the Locust).

Perform twice.

Unclasp hands and place chin in left hand. Fingers are together and rest on left cheek. Hold back of head firmly with right hand.

Use hands to slowly and firmly turn head as far as possible to left. Hold extreme position for a count of 10.

NOTES

In cases of exceptional stiffness or tension, each of the three positions may be held for up to a count of 60.

Be sure that your fingers are on the correct cheek. When you turn to the left (Figure 2), your fingers are on your left cheek; when you turn to the right, fingers are on right cheek.

Hold elbows parallel. If you allow them to spread, you will not have sufficient height.

Close your eyes during the movement and enjoy the feeling of neck tension dissolving. The Neck Movements can be done at any time of the day when quick relief from tension is required.

14
LOCUST

BENEFITS

Strengthens the entire body.

Firms arms, legs, lower abdomen, and buttocks.

Improves circulation.

With arms at sides, rest chin on mat. Make fists and place them thumbs down next to the thighs.

Tense all muscles. Push against the floor with fists and slowly raise left leg as high as possible. Bring the leg straight up and keep it steady.

Hold for a count of 10.

Slowly lower left leg to floor, and relax all muscles for a few moments.

Perform identical movements with right leg, holding extreme position for a count of 10.

Perform twice with each leg, alternating left and right.

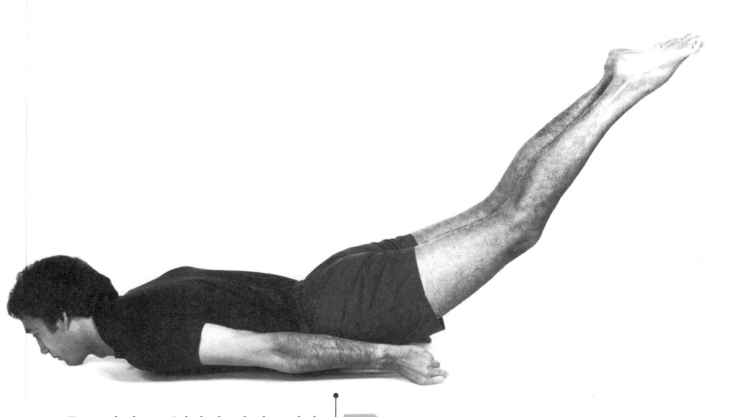

2

Empty the lungs. Inhale deeply through the nose and retain. Tense all muscles. Push hard against floor with fists and raise both legs, with knees together, as high as possible. Hold for a count of 5. Keep legs together; chin must not leave the floor.

Begin to exhale, and slowly lower legs to floor.

Relax all muscles for several moments. Inhale deeply, and repeat.

Perform twice.

NOTES

The deep inhalation will expand the chest and lend support to the lift.

In order to derive maximum benefits, lower legs slowly to the floor and exhale slowly; do not let breath gush from the lungs.

Be sure that sides of fists, not palms, press against the floor. Some students find that placing the fists nearer to the waist and bending the elbows allows for a higher lift.

As in all Yoga postures, the benefits are derived from performing the movements to the best of your ability, not from the immediate execution of an extreme position. Your proficiency in raising both legs will increase with regular practice. The results are well worth the efforts.

15

BOW

BENEFITS

Firms and strengthens back, spine, and thighs.

•

Develops and maintains flexibility.

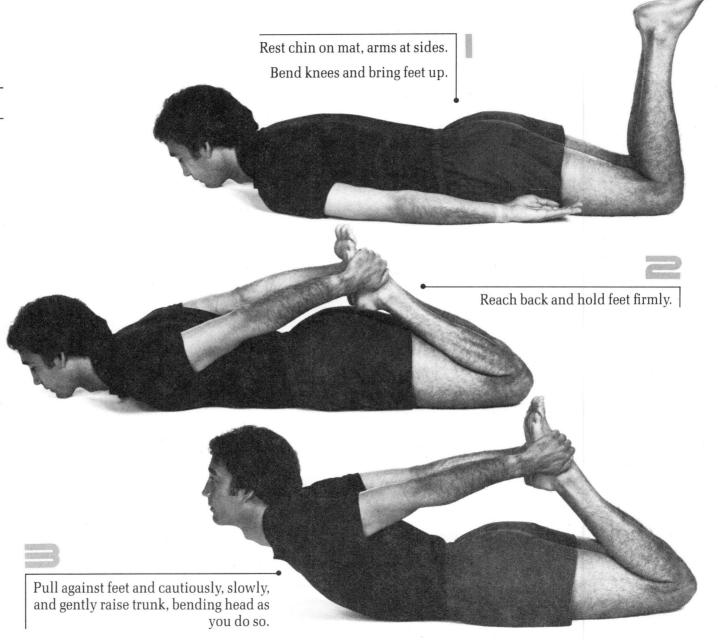

Rest chin on mat, arms at sides. **1**

Bend knees and bring feet up.

Reach back and hold feet firmly. **2**

3 Pull against feet and cautiously, slowly, and gently raise trunk, bending head as you do so.

Lower knees to floor *first*; then lower chin to floor but maintain hold on feet.

Rest several moments. Repeat.

Following final repetition, return knees and chin to floor; release feet and lower them slowly to floor. Rest cheek on floor, and relax completely.

Perform three times.

Continue to pull against feet and raise knees and thighs, raising trunk and legs as high as possible without strain.

Keep knees as close together as possible.

Hold for a count of 10.

4

NOTES

At first, you may have to struggle to hold both feet. Continued attempts will bring success. In your initial practice sessions you can hold one foot and then let go and try to hold the other. This practice will prepare you to hold both feet.

Raising the trunk (Figure 3) is not difficult, but raising knees and thighs (Figure 4) usually requires practice to develop the necessary muscle action.

Keeping the knees together during the raise places added emphasis on the spine. Holding the head back as far as possible during the raise aids in the spinal curvature.

In lowering (Figure 5) be sure that the chin is brought to the floor *first* and *then* lower the knees to the floor.

Proceed very cautiously, and never make any sudden or erratic movements. Practice to achieve slowness and control.

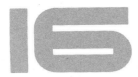

16
SIDE RAISE
BENEFITS

Firms legs, abdomen, buttocks and arms.

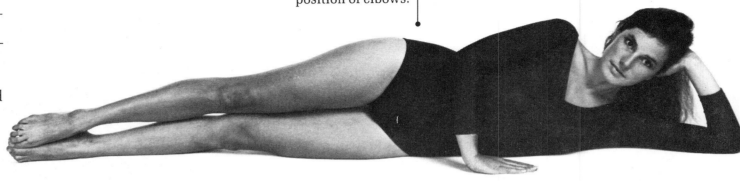

1 Lie on your left side with legs together, head supported by left hand, and right hand firmly on floor as illustrated. Note position of elbows.

2 Push down with right hand and raise legs together as high as possible.

Bring legs up directly from the side without swaying to front or back.

Hold as steady as possible for a count of 5.

Slowly lower legs to floor. Repeat.

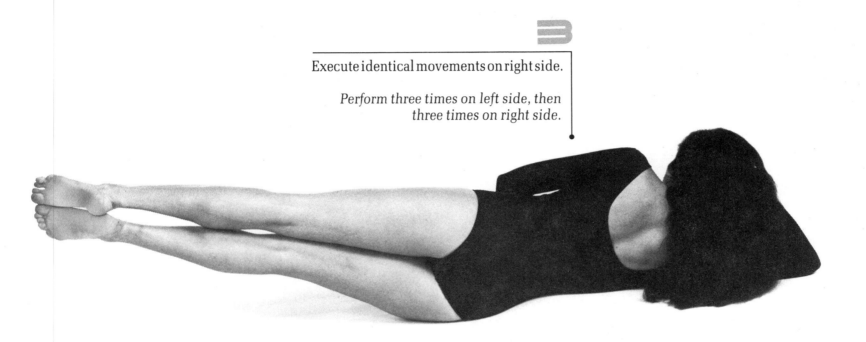

3

Execute identical movements on right side.

*Perform three times on left side, then
three times on right side.*

NOTES

For maximum benefits, be sure to
keep your legs together during the
lift and hold.

17
BACK
PUSH UP

BENEFITS

Firms and strengthens the entire body.

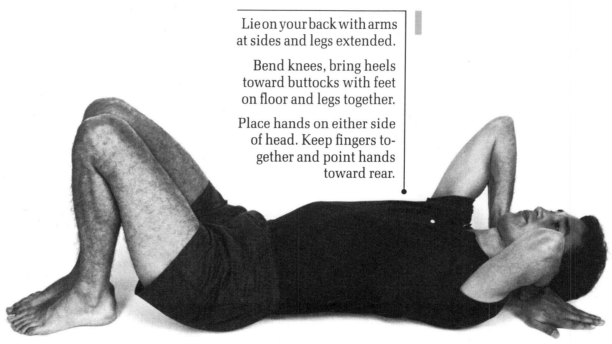

Lie on your back with arms at sides and legs extended.

Bend knees, bring heels toward buttocks with feet on floor and legs together.

Place hands on either side of head. Keep fingers together and point hands toward rear.

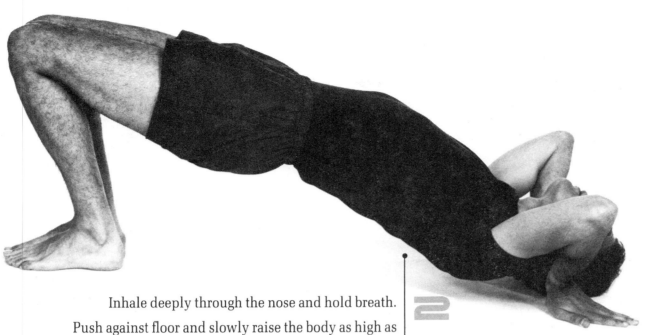

Inhale deeply through the nose and hold breath.

Push against floor and slowly raise the body as high as possible. As you raise, arch neck slightly to assist in lift.

Keep calves and knees together.

Hold for a count of 10.

Exhale through nose and simultaneously lower body slowly to floor. Repeat.

Following final repetition, slowly return arms to sides and extend legs.

Perform three times.

NOTES

Be sure that the palms of hands, not the fingertips, push against the floor.

Keeping the legs together increases the effectiveness of the movements.

Be cautious when arching the neck; do it slowly. When you feel ready, the top of the head can rest on the floor to increase the height of the lift.

18
SHOULDER STAND
BENEFITS

The benefits of the Shoulder Stand are too numerous to list or describe in detail. Briefly, it:

- Brings an increased supply of blood into the thyroid gland in the neck area, which often assists in weight normalization and redistribution;

- Aids in improving blood circulation in upper areas of body;

- Relaxes legs—very valuable for those who are constantly on their feet during the day;

- Relaxes various organs and glands that are continually subject to gravitational pull in the usual upright postion of the body.

1 Lie on back, arms at sides, palms on floor.

2 Stiffen leg and abdominal muscles; push against floor with hands and slowly raise legs, keeping knees straight.

3 Swing legs back over head.

Place hands firmly against lower back or hips.

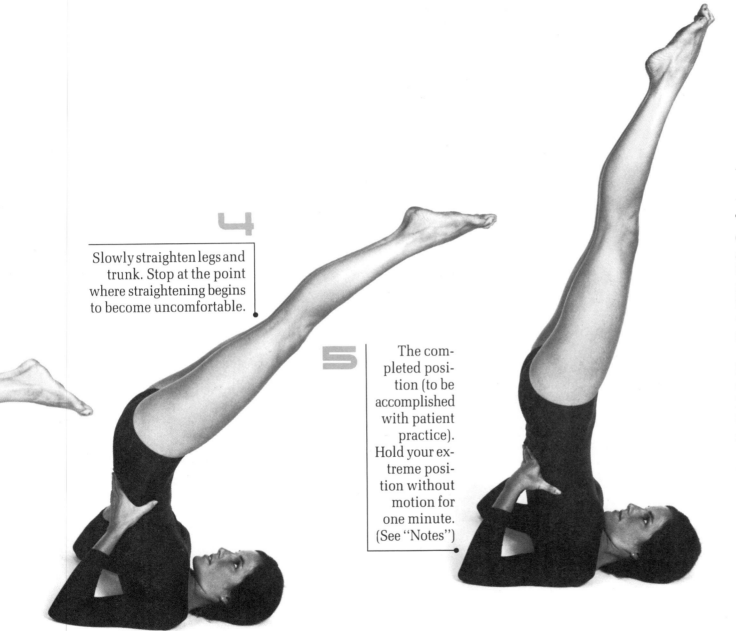

4

Slowly straighten legs and trunk. Stop at the point where straightening begins to become uncomfortable.

5

The completed position (to be accomplished with patient practice). Hold your extreme position without motion for one minute. (See "Notes")

NOTES

There is no hurry to attain the completed position of Figure 5. Any angle of inversion is of value. So even if you are able to accomplish only a very modified position of the Shoulder Stand, you will gradually be able to straighten to the extreme upright position.

Swinging the legs back over the head (Figure 3) assists in raising the lower back from the floor. If necessary, this movement can be done more quickly to gain momentum.

Begin the hold in your extreme position for one minute (or less, if necessary) and gradually add seconds until you have reached three minutes. Remain at three minutes length for several weeks, and when this has become entirely comfortable, you may, if you wish, continue to add seconds gradually until you have reached five or ten minutes. But increase the time

(Continued)

[41]

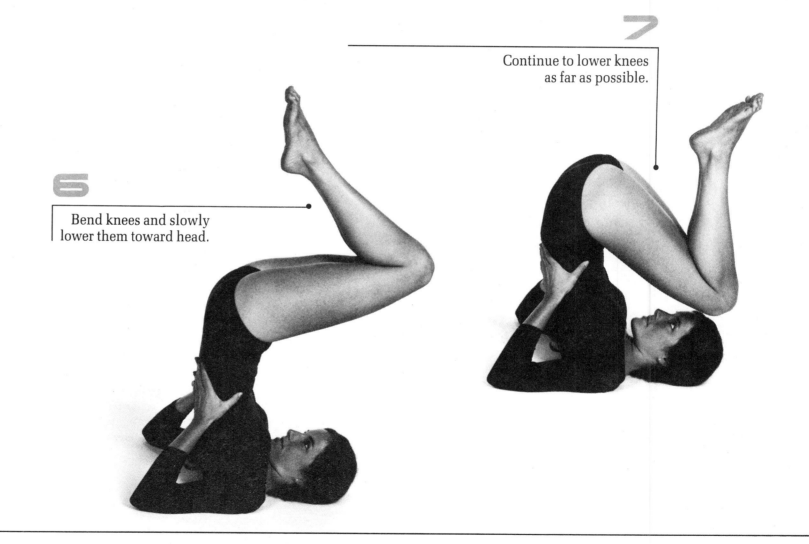

6 Bend knees and slowly lower them toward head.

7 Continue to lower knees as far as possible.

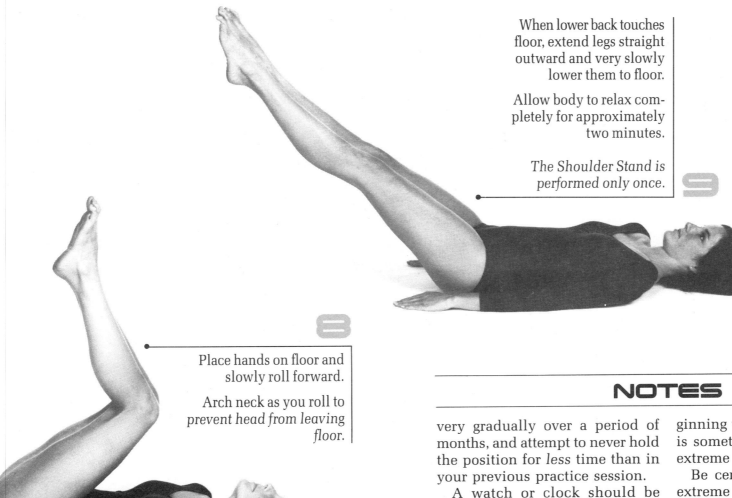

When lower back touches floor, extend legs straight outward and very slowly lower them to floor.

Allow body to relax completely for approximately two minutes.

The Shoulder Stand is performed only once.

9

8

Place hands on floor and slowly roll forward.

Arch neck as you roll to *prevent head from leaving floor.*

NOTES

very gradually over a period of months, and attempt to never hold the position for *less* time than in your previous practice session.

A watch or clock should be placed where it can be easily seen from the inverted position.

This extreme position should be held in a relaxed manner. There is no need to become tight or rigid.

Breathing should be slow and controlled.

A small pillow or folded towel placed under your neck before be-

ginning will relieve pressure that is sometimes experienced in the extreme position.

Be certain to come out of the extreme position *exactly as instructed* in Figures 6–9. These movements should flow into one another and be smooth and continuous.

When you have returned to the horizontal position and allowed the body to become limp, you will experience a deep relaxation and a subsequent revitalization.

19
PLOUGH
BENEFITS

Develops a high degree of spinal flexibility.

•

Extremely strengthening for the back.

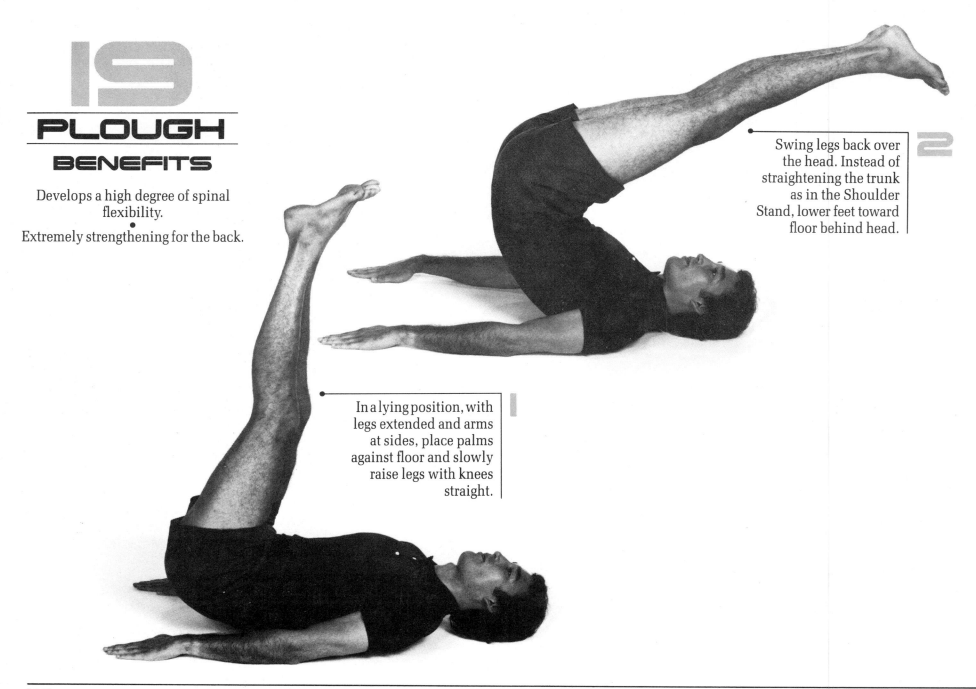

2 Swing legs back over the head. Instead of straightening the trunk as in the Shoulder Stand, lower feet toward floor behind head.

1 In a lying position, with legs extended and arms at sides, place palms against floor and slowly raise legs with knees straight.

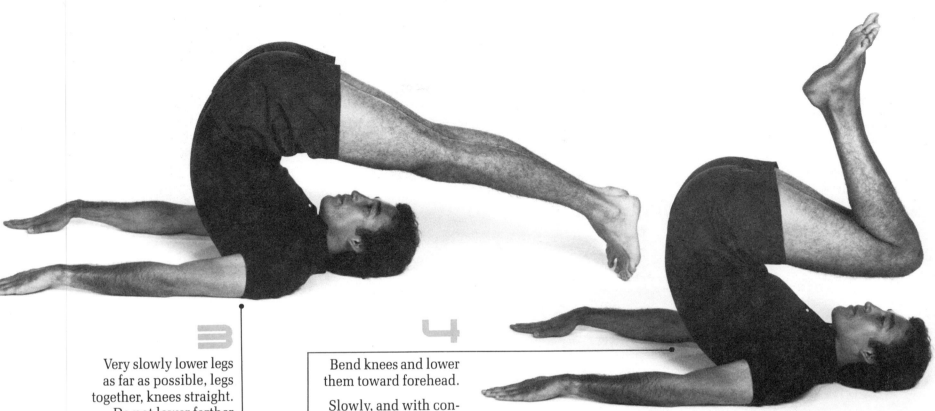

3

Very slowly lower legs as far as possible, legs together, knees straight. Do not lower farther than is comfortable. (Figure 3 depicts the extreme position, in which feet touch floor.)

Hold your extreme position for a count of 20.

4

Bend knees and lower them toward forehead.

Slowly, and with control, roll forward. When lower back touches floor, extend legs straight outward and very slowly lower them to floor.

Relax without movement for approximately thirty seconds. Repeat.

Perform twice.

NOTES

The advanced position of the Plough is accomplished by simply holding the extreme position and allowing the weight of the legs to gradually stretch the spine. Do not try to reach the extreme position by lunging backward or forcing the legs down. Increasing your stretch even an inch at a time over a period of weeks or months will strengthen each vertebra and help to develop lifelong flexibility.

With the chin pressed against the chest you may experience some difficulty in breathing. This can be overcome by focusing your attention on the respiration and making a point of breathing slowly and rhythmically.

20
COMPLETE
BREATH
BENEFITS

This technique imparts the many benefits inherent in breathing fully, deeply, and slowly. Such benefits include: improvement in the condition of the blood and its circulation, relief from physical and mental fatigue, revitalization, increase in lung capacity, and aid in respiratory conditions.

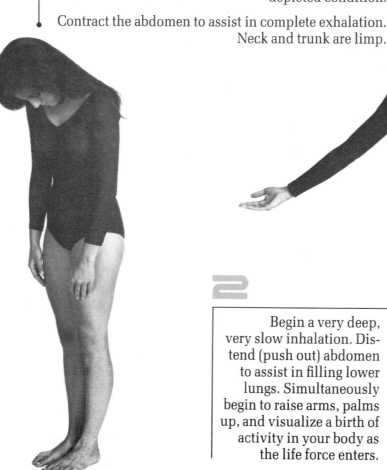

1 These movements are designed to assist in filling the lungs to capacity through very deep, slow inhalations *through the nose.*

With the feet several inches apart and arms at sides exhale deeply. As the breath (*prana,* life force) is expelled, there is a minimum of vitality. Feel and visualize this wilted, depleted condition.

Contract the abdomen to assist in complete exhalation. Neck and trunk are limp.

2 Begin a very deep, very slow inhalation. Distend (push out) abdomen to assist in filling lower lungs. Simultaneously begin to raise arms, palms up, and visualize a birth of activity in your body as the life force enters.

3

As you continue the deep, slow inhalation and slow rising of the arms, your chest expands, and you feel and visualize increased life force entering.

Now palms meet overhead, the lungs are filled, the chest fully expanded, maximum life force in the body. Feel and visualize this maximum condition.

Retain the air without moving for a count of 5.

4

Reverse the procedure: turn the palms outward and execute a very deep, slow exhalation through the nose, simultaneously lowering arms and contracting abdomen, until you have returned to position of Figure 1.

Repeat without pause.

Perform five times.

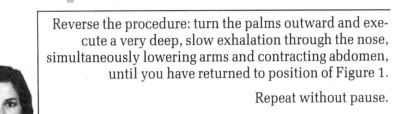

NOTES

Once begun, there is no interruption of the breathing. It is continuous throughout the five performances

You must inhale and exhale slowly enough to permit the coordination of the slow raising and lowering of the arms with your breathing.

The Complete Breath can be performed in almost any situation that requires clearing of the mind or overcoming a negative emotion, or simple revitalization. In a seated posture you would modify the technique by eliminating the arms movement. When possible, fold hands in lap and close eyes.

Now that you have become familiar with the type of movements and holds that comprise the *Hatha* Yoga system, you can undertake the following three essential techniques. These are comparatively more difficult because of the muscular control, balance, and flexibility that are required.

You can consider these movements and postures as more advanced *Hatha* Yoga, and let them serve as challenges for future months of practice. As you continue the *Hatha* Yoga program, you will find that your body will develop the strength and capability for advancing to the more difficult positions. You will be able to determine for yourself when you are ready to attempt these three advanced exercises, but always be guided by the principle of never doing more than is comfortable, and *never strain*.

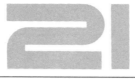

21
ABDOMINAL LIFT

BENEFITS

Tones the abdominal muscles.

•

Stimulates organs of the viscera and aids the peristaltic action.

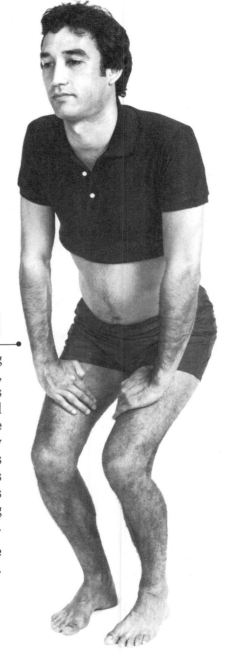

In a standing position, bend knees several inches, place hands firmly on thighs with fingers and thumbs pointing inward.

Relax the abdomen.

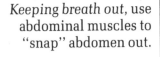

3

Keeping breath out, use abdominal muscles to "snap" abdomen out.

Without pause, and *keeping air out of lungs,* repeat.

Perform five lifts, *allowing no air to enter the lungs.*

Following fifth lift, inhale slowly, and straighten trunk to upright position. Bring arms to sides, and breathe normally for several moments.

Return body to position of Figure 1. Repeat.

Perform five rounds (twenty-five lifts).

2

Exhale very deeply through the nose and empty the lungs completely.

Keeping breath out, push down on thighs with hands and, *without inhaling,* lift or "suck in" abdomen.

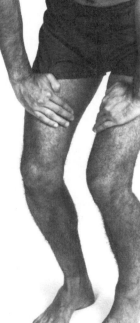

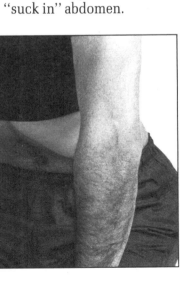

NOTES

In order to lift the abdomen, it is necessary to create a type of "vacuum" by emptying the lungs and keeping them empty. Therefore, a deep, complete exhalation is essential.

In the beginning, you may be able to only contract the abdomen and not execute the complete lift. This is perfectly satisfactory, because as you gain control of the abdominal muscles, the contraction is transformed into the lift.

The "snapping out" of Figure 3 is a forceful movement of the abdominal muscles. Do not permit the abdomen to simply relax, but "pop" or "shoot" it out.

When five lifts become easy, you can increase the number to ten or more lifts to each exhalation and perform a total of fifty to one hundred lifts in the practice session.

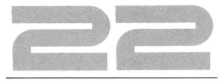

22
HEAD
STAND

BENEFITS

Increases supply of blood into head. It thereby:

• Refreshes brain, helping to prevent hardening of arteries and symptoms of senility;

• Improves condition of face, scalp, and hair;

• Assists in the maintenance and improvement of vision and hearing;

• Reverses gravitational pressure on glands and organs (including heart).

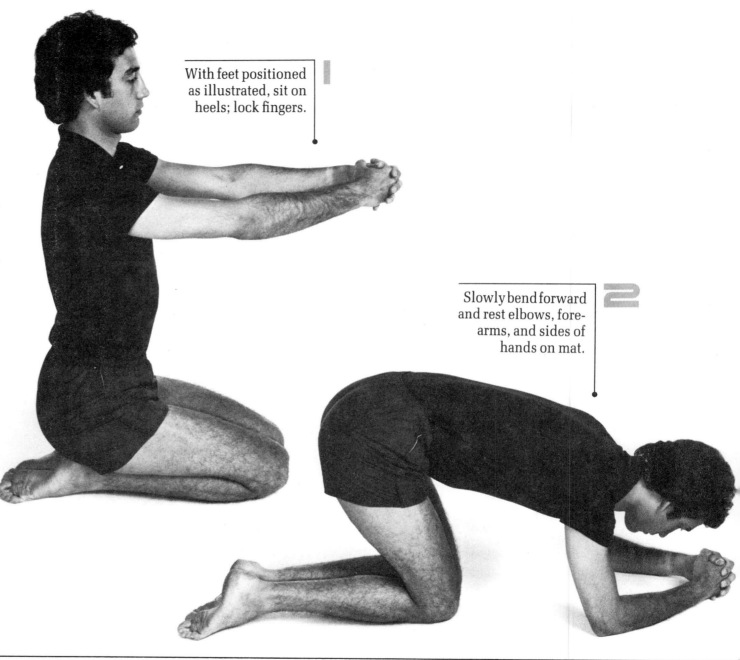

1 With feet positioned as illustrated, sit on heels; lock fingers.

2 Slowly bend forward and rest elbows, forearms, and sides of hands on mat.

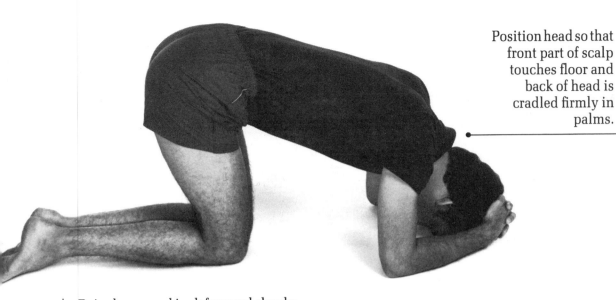

Position head so that front part of scalp touches floor and back of head is cradled firmly in palms.

3

In Figure 3, be sure that the hands are not simply lying on the floor. The fingers are tightly locked together, the sides of the hands rest firmly on the floor and the palms have a secure grip on the *back* of the head.

The closer you can bring your knees to your chest (Figure 4), the easier it will be to perform the next stage of the Head Stand.

Direct contact between your head and the mat or floor may prove uncomfortable. If so, place a small pillow or folded towel beneath your head to decrease the pressure on head and neck.

During your first few attempts of the position of Figure 5, you may experience some discomfort as the blood flows more rapidly into your head. This feeling of increased pressure should disappear within one to two weeks of practice.

Gradually increase the duration of your holds in the extreme positions from thirty seconds to the indicated maximum. Add approximately ten to twenty seconds per week. Either approximate seconds in your mental counting, or place a timepiece where it may be easily seen.

(Continued)

4

Raise knees and inch forward slowly with toes until knees are as close to chest as possible. Do not straighten knees.

Hold thirty to sixty seconds.

Slowly and gently lower knees to floor.

Slowly raise head and gradually return to a seated position. Relax.

Do not go beyond this position during the first two weeks of your practice of this exercise.

This elementary position is performed once.

Following the first two weeks of practice:

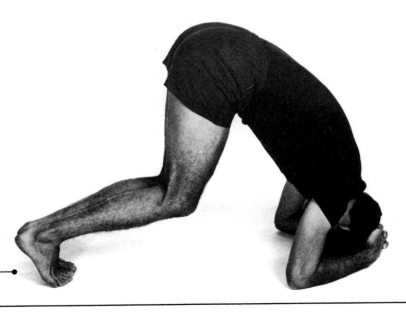

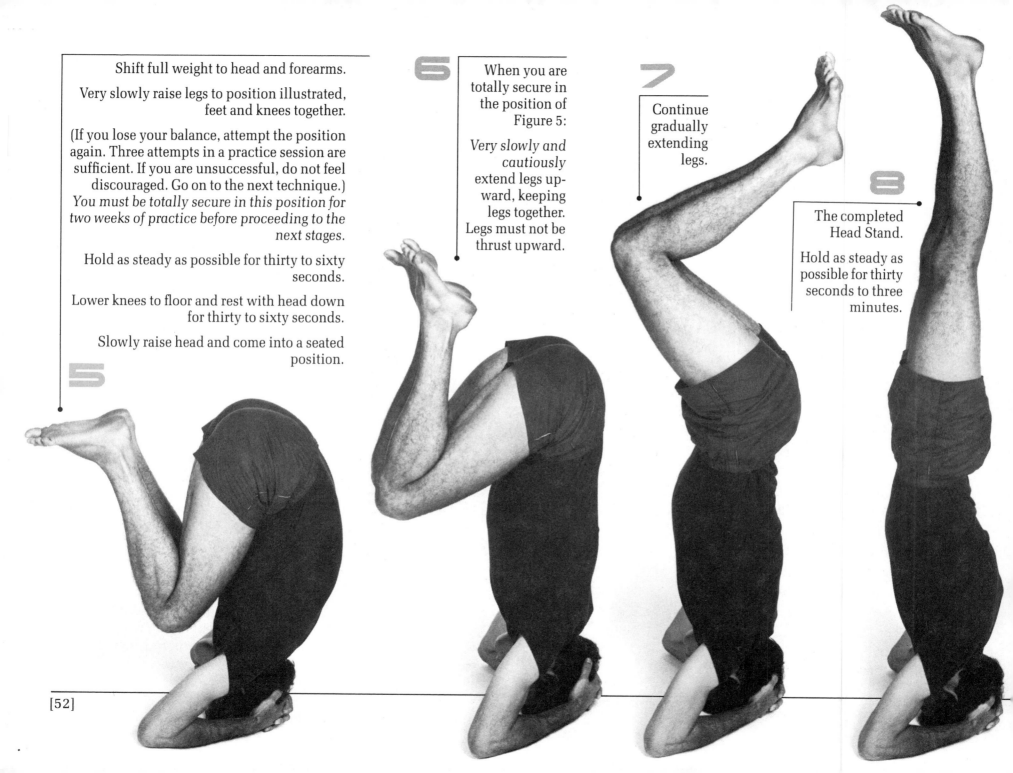

5

Shift full weight to head and forearms.

Very slowly raise legs to position illustrated, feet and knees together.

(If you lose your balance, attempt the position again. Three attempts in a practice session are sufficient. If you are unsuccessful, do not feel discouraged. Go on to the next technique.) *You must be totally secure in this position for two weeks of practice before proceeding to the next stages.*

Hold as steady as possible for thirty to sixty seconds.

Lower knees to floor and rest with head down for thirty to sixty seconds.

Slowly raise head and come into a seated position.

6

When you are totally secure in the position of Figure 5:

Very slowly and cautiously extend legs upward, keeping legs together. Legs must not be thrust upward.

7

Continue gradually extending legs.

8

The completed Head Stand.

Hold as steady as possible for thirty seconds to three minutes.

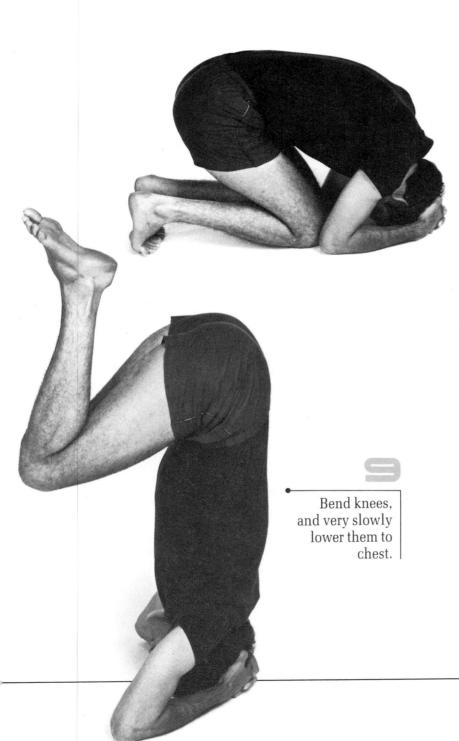

Touch toes to floor and remain with head down for thirty to sixty seconds.

Slowly raise head and come into a seated position.

Perform once. (If you lose balance, make one or two additional attempts. If unsuccessful do not feel discouraged. Go on to next technique.)

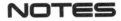

10

9

Bend knees, and very slowly lower them to chest.

NOTES

Carefully note the word "slowly" as it appears in the directions. If you catch yourself beginning to move too quickly, change that movement into slow motion.

Never jump up suddenly when you have completed the exercise. A sudden change can make you dizzy. Always rest with head down, as indicated. Persons with high blood pressure or cardiac conditions should check with their physicians regarding the Head Stand and always proceed cautiously.

It is most important to not become impatient in attempting to reach the extreme upright positions. If you are not secure in the position of Figure 5, you should not go on. You must have control in each of the movements or you will not fully benefit from the Head Stand and you will never truly gain the necessary balance.

Some students use the wall as an aid during their initial practice. The body is placed close to the wall and it supports the back and legs in Figures 5–8. However, you should not resort to the wall until you have attempted the movements many times and are absolutely convinced that you are not making progress.

Surround yourself with a few pillows for added protection in the event that you lose your balance.

Do not give up even if your progress is slow. Tens of thousands of Yoga students beyond middle age who in their entire lives had never inverted their bodies have accomplished the completed Head Stand with patient practice.

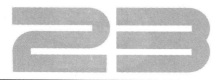

LOTUS POSTURES

BENEFITS

Promotes flexibility of the knees, ankles, and feet.

•

Develops the ability to remain firmly and quietly seated for periods of meditation.

This is the Simple Seated Pose. **I**

Sides of feet should rest on floor as depicted. At first, if it's easier, ankles may be crossed with knees raised.

Hold spine and head straight, but relaxed.

Rest backs of hands on knees, and touch index fingers to thumbs. Lower eyelids.

Preparation for the Half Lotus: **2**

Extend both legs.

Using both hands, place left heel as far in as possible.

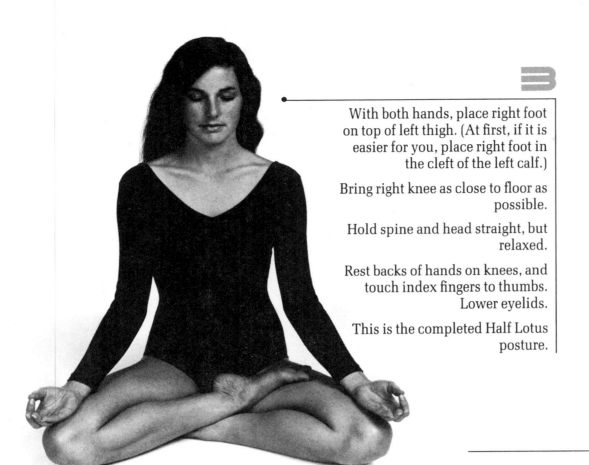

3

With both hands, place right foot on top of left thigh. (At first, if it is easier for you, place right foot in the cleft of the left calf.)

Bring right knee as close to floor as possible.

Hold spine and head straight, but relaxed.

Rest backs of hands on knees, and touch index fingers to thumbs. Lower eyelids.

This is the completed Half Lotus posture.

NOTES

Assume whichever of the three postures is comfortable. As the necessary flexibility is developed, the knees will automatically lower and the more advanced Lotus positions can be attained.

A small pillow that provides approximately six inches of sitting height can be used. This additional height raises the trunk and simul-taneously lowers the knees. However, if the postures present no difficulty, the pillow need not be used.

In both the Half and Full Lotus postures, practice by placing first one foot on top and then, as that position becomes uncomfortable, stretch the legs out for a few

(Continued)

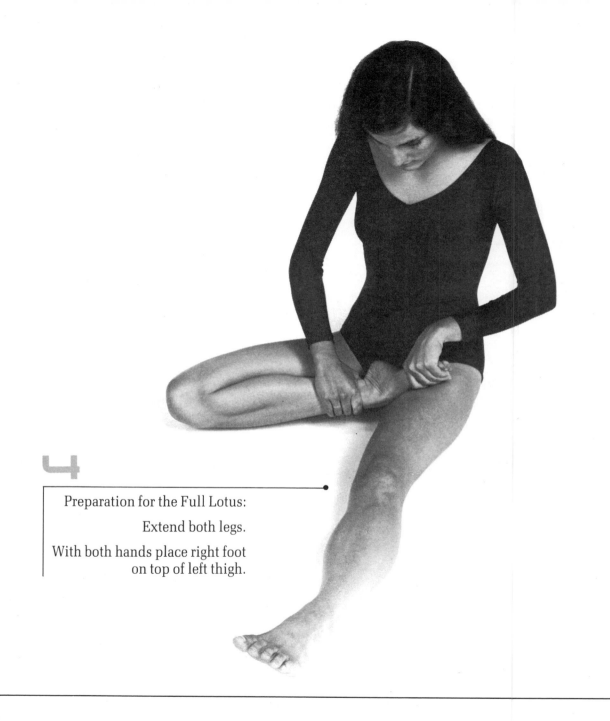

4

Preparation for the Full Lotus:

Extend both legs.

With both hands place right foot
on top of left thigh.

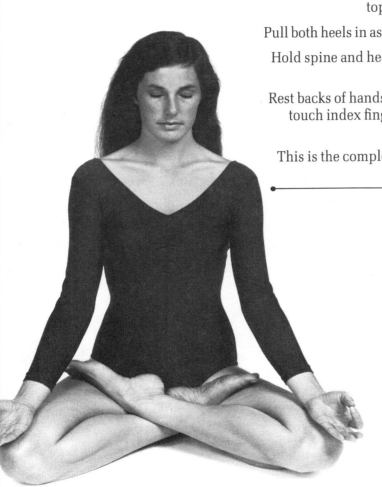

With both hands place left foot on top of right thigh.

Pull both heels in as far as possible.

Hold spine and head straight, but relaxed.

Rest backs of hands on knees, and touch index fingers to thumbs. Lower eyelids.

This is the completed Full Lotus posture.

5

NOTES

moments and reverse their position. But practice to eventually attain those positions of the legs indicated in the photographs, because they are traditional for meditation.

The eyes are not entirely closed. A slit of light is allowed to enter at the bottom. In this manner you remain suspended between the waking and sleeping states.

Touching the index fingers to the thumbs closes the circuit of energy and keeps the life force within the body.

Assume one of the Lotus postures for Alternate Nostril Breathing, the Special Routine, and all meditation practices.

24

SPECIAL
ROUTINE

BENEFITS

This is a simple group of movements designed to manipulate areas of the body that are frequently neglected in ordinary exercising.

These pulls and stretches reach into tension areas, loosen joints and muscles, relieve fatigue, and replenish energy.

1

Sit in a Lotus posture for the entire routine.

Firmly hold right thumb with left hand, pull hard as though you would stretch the thumb, and hold the pull for a count of 2.

Pull index finger and hold for a count of 2. Pull each of the remaining three fingers in turn.

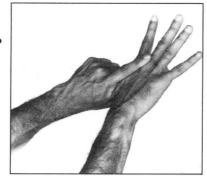

2

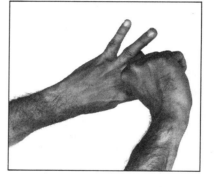

Execute identical movements with fingers of the left hand.

Perform only once with each finger.

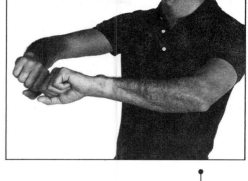

Make fists of the hands and position arms as illustrated.

3

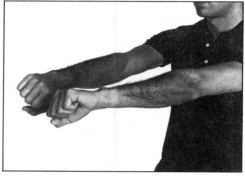

4

In a quick, forceful movement, snap arms outward until elbows are straight.

Hold straightened position of arms for a count of 2.

Return arms to position of Figure 3. Repeat.

Perform ten times.

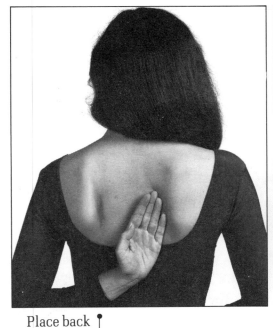

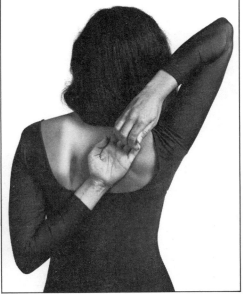

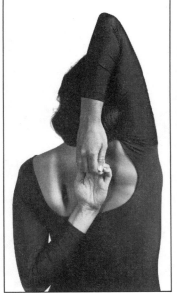

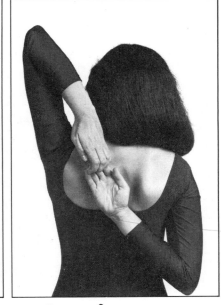

Place back
of left hand
against upper
back.

Bring right
hand over
back so that
fingers of
hands can
clasp one
another.

5

Slowly and
gently, pull
up with right
arm so that
left arm is
raised one to
two inches.

Hold for a
count of 5.

6

Slowly and
gently, pull
down with
left arm so
that right is
lowered one
to two inches.

Hold for a
count of 5.

Trunk re-
mains erect;
do not slump.

*Perform the
upward and
downward
pulls three
times.*

7

Reverse
position of
arms and
execute iden-
tical move-
ments three
times.

Return hands
to knees.

8

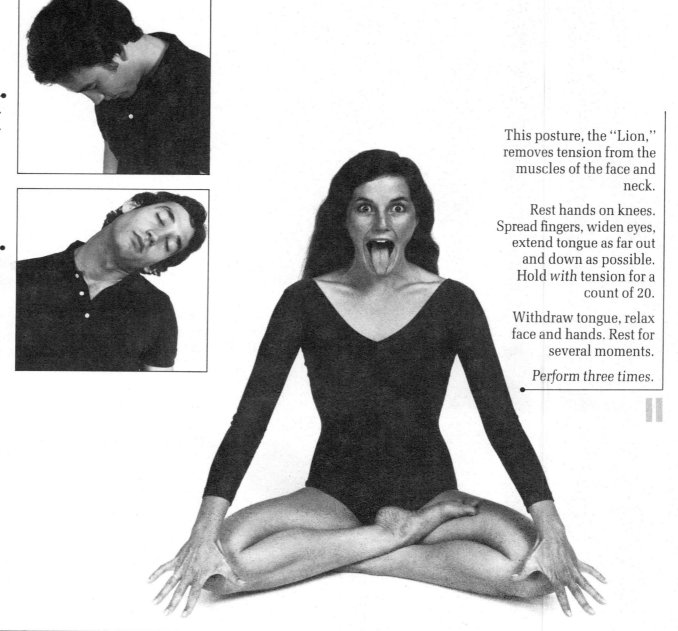

Close eyes and rest chin on chest. Hold this position for a count of 5.

10. In very slow motion, *roll and twist* head to extreme left. Hold for a count of 5.

Very slowly, roll and twist head to extreme backward position. Feel skin of chin and throat tighten. Hold for a count of 5.

Keep trunk erect throughout movements. Do not slump or move trunk forward or backward.

Very slowly roll and twist head to extreme right position . Hold for a count of 5.

Be sure that head is not simply bending into the positions, but that it is rolling and twisting.

Very slowly roll and twist head to forward position of Figure 9.

Perform three times.

This posture, the "Lion," removes tension from the muscles of the face and neck.

Rest hands on knees. Spread fingers, widen eyes, extend tongue as far out and down as possible. Hold *with* tension for a count of 20.

Withdraw tongue, relax face and hands. Rest for several moments.

Perform three times.

11

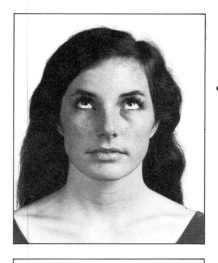

 12

Widen eye sockets and hold them this way throughout these movements.

Slowly move eyes to tops of sockets. Hold for one second.

 13

Slowly *roll* eyes to extreme right position; to bottom position; to extreme left position.

Hold each position for one second.

Roll eyes to top position and repeat.

Perform ten rounds.

Close eyes and rest them for several moments.

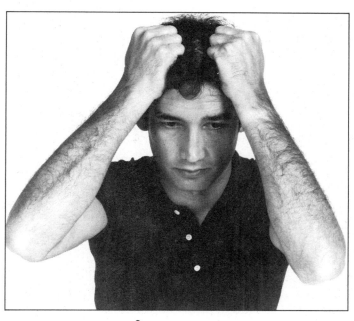

 15

Pull vigorously and make scalp move first foreward, then backward.

Perform twenty-five forward and backward movements, rhythmically but not too quickly.

(Hands may also be moved to other areas of scalp if a total massage is desired. Perform twenty-five times in each area.

Reach down deeply into roots of hair and firmly grasp as much hair as you can hold with both hands.

14

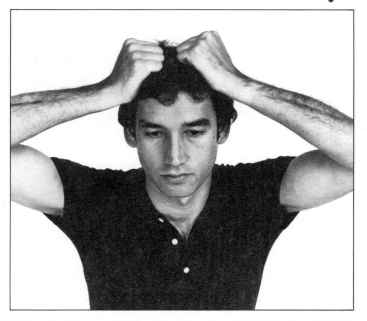

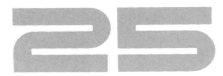

25
DEEP RELAXATION
BENEFITS

Imparts a state of total physical, mental, and emotional relaxation.

Deep Relaxation, Alternate Nostril Breathing, and Directing the Life Force are three classical relaxation-meditation techniques. One of the three will be utilized as the final technique of each practice session.

The objective of this technique is to place the body, mind, and emotions in a state of total serenity. You may believe that by lying as depicted in the photograph and simply relaxing, you can attain this tranquil condition. But it is usually the case that you will be experiencing tensions and muscular contractions of which you are not even aware, and the mind continues to race at its customary frantic pace. This is not *total* relaxation. To achieve *total* relaxation, undertake the procedure described below.

Lying on your back with arms at sides, adjust the body into its most comfortable position.

We want to become aware of each area of the body to determine if it is truly relaxed (limp). Begin by directing full attention to the feet. If tensed in any way, relax them.

Next, focus attention on the calves and knees. "Feel" them with your consciousness, and

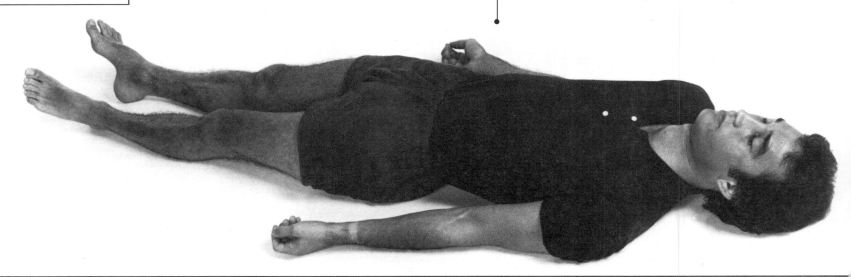

remove all tension by making the necessary adjustments. Slowly draw the consciousness into the lower abdomen, upper abdomen, chest. If you detect even the slightest muscular contraction, relax it.

Now become aware of the fingers, forearms, upper arms, and shoulders. "Feel" the condition of each of these, and withdraw all support so that it becomes limp. Adjust the neck as necessary, and relax jaw and all facial muscles.

If you know yourself to be an exceptionally tense person, repeat the entire procedure.

Finally, direct your attention to your breathing. Have it become slow and rhythmic. This will minimize the thoughts that can enter and divert the mind.

You are now in a state of profound relaxation. Remain this way for several minutes with the attention fully focused on your breathing.

NOTES

As you continue to practice this technique, you will be able to achieve the total relaxation state more and more quickly, and the depth of the relaxation will continue to increase. Once you get the feeling of the deeply relaxed condition, you will be able to attain it in a sitting or even a standing position. The technique becomes applicable whenever necessary during the workday.

26
ALTERNATE NOSTRIL BREATHING
BENEFITS

Acts as a profound natural tranquilizer, providing relief from mental and emotional tension and fatigue.

Assists in clearing the nasal passages.

Highly effective in eliminating tension headaches.

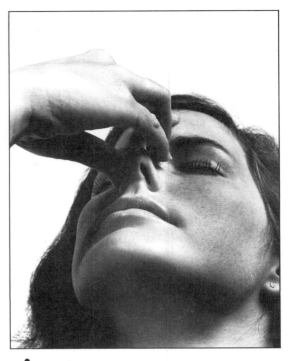

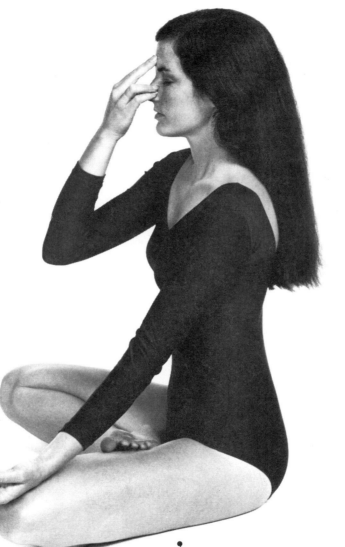

Exhale fully.

Press right nostril closed with thumb. Inhale through the left nostril and fill the lungs during a slow, rhythmic count of 8.

2

Sit in a Lotus posture and place hand as illustrated. Once the directions are learned, close your eyes during the entire exercise.

1

4

Open the *right* nostril (the left remains closed), and exhale fully during a rhythmic count of 8.

Without pause:

Inhale through the *right* nostril (the same nostril through which you just exhaled) during a rhythmic count of 8.

Close the *right* nostril (both nostrils are now closed) and retain for a count of 4.

Open the *left* nostril (the right remains closed) and exhale fully during a count of 8.

This completes one round. *Without pause,* repeat by inhaling through the *left* nostril, etc.

Perform five rounds.

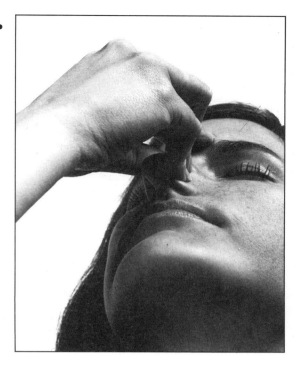

3

Close the left nostril with the ring and little fingers so that both nostrils are now closed.

Retain the air for a rhythmic count of 4.

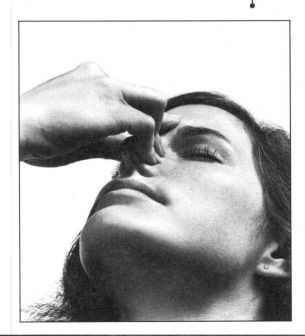

NOTES

Breathe quietly and deeply.

Keep the hands relaxed, the spine straight, and the head raised.

Maintain the rhythmic count of 8-4-8; 8-4-8. Do not interrupt this rhythm. Here is a summary of the technique:

Exhale deeply

Inhale through left _____ Count 8
Retain (both closed) _____ Count 4
Exhale through right _____ Count 8

Inhale through right _____ Count 8
Retain (both closed) _____ Count 4
Exhale through left _____ Count 8

This completes one round.

You can practice this breathing technique at any time of the day when you wish to calm your emotions, withdraw your mind and senses from external activities, and become aware of your spiritual reality.

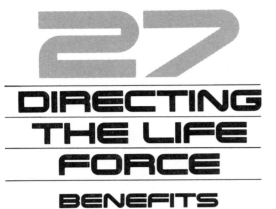

27
DIRECTING THE LIFE FORCE

BENEFITS

Elevates the consciousness.
•
Can be utilized as a healing exercise.

Lie on your back. Close eyes and relax deeply.

Place all fingers on solar plexus. During a slow, quiet inhalation through the nose, visualize an intense white light being drawn from your solar plexus into fingertips.

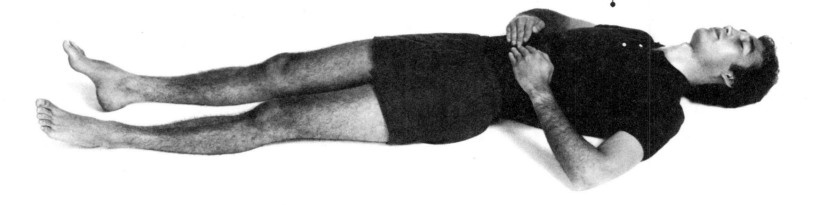

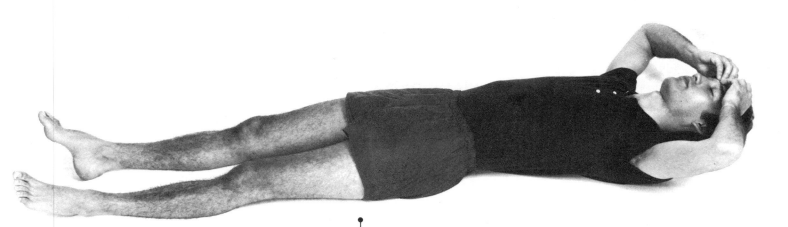

When the inhalation is completed, retain air, and transfer fingertips to forehead.

During a slow, quiet exhalation, visualize the same white light flowing from your fingertips into your head. The entire area surrounding your head is permeated in brilliant illumination.

When exhalation is completed, return fingertips to solar plexus and repeat without pause.

Perform seven rounds. This technique can be applied whenever necessary.

2

NOTES

Some people have difficulty in visualizing the white light; either they cannot see it at all, or it appears and fades. To visualize continually requires full concentration, what in Yoga is designated as "one-pointedness." To achieve this you must practice. Acquiring the ability to focus your attention in this "one-pointed" manner will be of great value to you not only in Yoga, but in all of your activities.

When utilizing this technique for healing purposes, the inhalation is the same as described in the directions, but during the exhalation the fingertips are placed on the afflicted area. You then visualize the white light flowing into and illuminating the area involved. If the problem lies in the legs or back, the technique should be performed in one of the Lotus postures so that the hands can reach the pertinent area during the exhalation.

If you find that it is absolutely impossible to visualize the white light, simply place your full attention on the breathing during both the inhalation and exhalation.

It is essential to keep your mind clear; consequently, you must be alert to any thoughts that begin to arise. Gently banish such distractions and return your total attention to the visualization or the breathing.

PRACTICE PLAN

All of the Yoga exercises presented in this section are included in the three routines on the opposite page. By rotating these routines (one routine for each day's practice session of thirty to forty minutes), you will be practicing all of the exercises over a period of three days. For example, on Monday, do Routine 1; Tuesday, do Routine 2; Wednesday, do Routine 3; Thursday, do Routine 1; etc. If you miss a day of practice, pick up where you left off. That is, if you performed Routine 2 on Tuesday and missed practice on Wednesday, on Thursday you would perform Routine 3.

If you practice with the Yoga For Health television programs, you will use these routines for additional practice at another time of the day, or when the programs are not seen.

You must continue to refer to the "Directions" of each exercise until you are *thoroughly familiar* with its correct execution, holding time and number of repetitions.

If you become very serious, and if your time permits, you may perform one entire routine earlier in the day and another entire routine later the same day. But continue to rotate the routines.

If absolutely necessary, you may divide a routine into two parts, practicing one part earlier in the day and the other at a later time.

Each routine begins with the Complete Breath and terminates with a relaxation-meditation technique. The routines are in standing-sitting-lying order.

ROUTINE I

20. Complete Breath
(p.46)

1. Chest Expansion
(p.6)

5. Roll Twist
(p.14)

9. Back Stretch
(p.22)

8. Twist
(p.20)

12. Cobra
(p.28)

13. Neck Movements
(p. 30)

14. Locust
(p. 32)

15. Bow
(p. 34)

25. Deep Relaxation
(p. 62)

ROUTINE 2

20. Complete Breath
    (p. 46)

3. Rishi's Posture
   (p. 10)

6. Dancer's Posture
   (p. 16)

21. Abdominal Lift
    (p. 48)

11. Backward Bend
    (p. 26)

10. Alternate Leg Stretch
    (p. 24)

19. Plough
    (p. 44)

22. Head Stand
    (p. 50)

26. Alternate Nostril Breathing
    (p. 64)

ROUTINE 3

20. Complete Breath
    (p. 46)

2. Triangle
   (p. 8)

4. Balance Posture
   (p. 12)

7. Knee and Thigh Stretch
   (p. 18)

24. Special Routine
    (p. 58)

16. Side Raise
    (p. 36)

17. Back Push Up
    (p. 38)

18. Shoulder Stand
    (p. 40)

27. Directing the Life Force
    (p. 66)

YOGA FOR PROBLEMS

Various physical and emotional problems have frequently responded in a highly favorable manner to Yoga practice. Those techniques that can aid in achieving certain objectives, or be applied to particular problems are indicated on the following pages. These are not suggested as an alternative to professional treatment; rather, with the physician's approval, they offer a form of physical therapy that can work to great advantage in conjunction with the general treatment that has been prescribed.

In electing to apply any of these "problem" routines, you must not neglect to perform the entire program of practice as presented in the Practice Plan (unless otherwise directed by your physician). You devote additional time to the indicated techniques either by increasing the number of repetitions during the course of your regular practice, or by performing *only* the "problem" routines(s) at another time of the day.

ABODOMEN

Strengthened, firmed, raised: Exercises 21, 14, 18, 19.

ARMS

Including shoulders and hands; firmed, strengthened: Exercises 1, 2, 24 (fingers, shoulders) 17, 14, 22.

ARTHRITIS

The slow motion movements and "holds" of the Yoga exercises have provided relief for the arthritis victim. With the approval of the physician, all of the less demanding techniques can be undertaken in a modified manner. The movements can be limited to a few inches and the "holds" maintained for only a few seconds each. This type of self-manipulation, in conjunction with the application of the Yoga dietary principles, offers the possibility of effective therapy for those suffering from this painful condition.

BACK

All areas strengthened, firmed; stiffness and tension relieved: Exercises 1, 3, 8, 12, 14, 15, 9, 19.

BALANCE

Exercises 3, 4, 6, 18, 22.

BLOOD

Circulation improved; pressure regulated: Exercises 20, 1, 3, 12, 14, 18, 19, 22.

CHEST

Expanded, developed; bust firmed, developed: Exercises 1, 4, 12, 15, 11.

CONSTIPATION

Exercise 21.

FEET

Including ankles and toes; strengthened, stiffness relieved: Exercises 6, 11, 23.

HEADACHES

Exercises 26, 27, 25, 20, 18, 19.

LEGS

Thighs and calves firmed, strengthened, and developed; tension relieved: Exercises 2, 6, 10, 14, 15, 19, 11, 18.

LUNGS

Cleansed, capacity increased: Exercises: 20, 1, 26.

MENSTRUATION

Practice during menstruation varies widely among students. Some do not wish to exercise, but many have found that the discomfort of the period is reduced through practice of the milder stretching, breathing, and inverted positions. You will have to experiment to determine what is best for you.

NECK

Strengthened; tension, stiffness relieved: Exercises 13, 24 (neck), 2, 3, 8, 11.

NERVOUS SYSTEM

General tension and insomnia relieved: Exercises 20, 1, 12, 13, 8, 9, 18, 26, 25.

POSTURE

Exercises 1, 11, 12, 15, 24 (Hand Clasp).

PREGNANCY

With the approval of the physician, moderate positions of the following can be performed during pregnancy: Exercises 2, 6, 9, 7, 8, 11, 16. Also, breathing exercises 20, 26.

POSTNATAL: See ABDOMEN.

RESPIRATORY CONDITIONS

The entire Yoga exercise program, performed in conjunction with the dietary principles.

SCALP, HAIR

Exercises 22, 24 (Scalp).

SPINE

Vertebrae manipulated; stiffness and tension relieved: Exercises for back.

WEIGHT

Regulation and maintenance, in conjunction with the dietary principles; waist and hips: Exercises 5, 21, 2, 8, 18, 19; buttocks, thighs, and calves: Exercises 2, 3, 6, 12, 14, 15, 16, 17, 18.

PART 2
NUTRITION

INTRODUCTION

The study and practice of Yoga are designed to enable each individual to develop his or her full potential; that is, to experience self-realization. The Yoga nutrition principles constitute an essential aspect of the program. Application of these principles will increase the benefits of the exercises. Anyone seeking to develop or regain health of body and mind must, sooner or later, recognize the indispensable role that is played by nutrition in this endeavor. The Yoga concept of "life-force" nutrition is as valid and effective today as when it was taught by the *Gurus* in ancient times.

The subtle element that sustains life is known in Yoga as *prana*; this can be translated as "life-force." (In Part IV of this book the concept of life-force is explained in detail.) All living organisms must have a steady and abundant supply of life-force. If the supply is inadequate, irregular, or unbalanced, the quality of life will suffer accordingly. In Yoga, we consider many physical, emotional, and mental disorders in terms of irregularities in the supply of life-force. When life-force falls below levels necessary to maintain good health, your body makes certain compensations. For example, you might feel a need for more sleep, or to eat more, or less, or even to fast. If you pay attention to these signals, you can maintain a good level of health. If you ignore them, as people too often do, you will suffer negative consequences in varying degrees.

It is generally recognized today that the average American diet is too high in fats, salts, and refined sugars. We eat more protein than we really need, and too few complex carbohydrates. Highly "advanced" processing techniques have robbed foods of many of their nutrients, and chemical additives, designed to prolong shelf life of foods in supermarkets, have often been shown to be harmful. The fact that one eats a five-, six-, or seven-course meal does not necessarily mean that one is being nourished. (Rather, it may be a testimonial to the incredible strength and recuperative powers of the body that it can absorb this abuse three times a day, year after year, and still survive!) We believe that many of the health problems associated with old age (and even earlier) can be attributed to years of imprudent and excess eating, as well as a lack of body conditioning.

Through the Yoga program of eating for maximum nutritional value, we believe it is possible to reverse the course of many of these problems, regenerate the organism, and prevent future "breakdowns." This is accomplished by activating the life-force that is currently present but repressed within the organism, by increasing the supply of life-force from external sources (air and food), and by eliminating or minimizing those activities and substances that inhibit or reduce the life-force, so that it is maintained at its optimum level. It must be clearly understood, however, that our concern with the life-force is not only for purposes of restoration of health and prevention of illness. The increased *prana* derived from *Hatha* Yoga and Yoga nutrition can serve to elevate the consciousness and direct the mind into fruitful meditation. To serious Yogis, these are of primary importance.

The guiding principles of Yoga nutrition emerge from the concept of eating foods that grow, foods in their natural state. They can be expressed in four basic questions: How much life-force is in this food? If not in its natural state, to what degree has it been altered? Is it easy for me to digest? What method of preparation will least decrease its nutritional value? The following pages contain information that will help you answer these questions.

In Yoga nutrition, the most desirable foods are fruits, vegetables, nuts, seeds, and certain grains. When eaten in as natural a state as digestion will permit, they provide the high quality of life-force that Yoga students seek. But remember that when these foods—as well as flesh, milk, and eggs—are refined, canned, preserved, boiled, frozen, smoked, aged, colored, fumigated, bleached, emulsified, thickened and otherwise processed, they are greatly reduced in nutritional value and life-force.

At this point it may seem that we are going to advise you to restrict your diet in the usual unpleasant way that requires waging a constant battle between what you think you really *want* to eat and what you *should* eat. It is not our intention to deprive you of the fun of eating, but to have you experience that eating for maximum Yoga nutritional value can be more satisfying and far more rewarding than your present diet.

In the past you may have been unsuccessful in attempts to eliminate from your diet foods that you know aren't good for you. Even if you succeeded for a while, your resolve eventually may have broken down and you resorted to your old habits. These failures were due to the fact that you were not totally convinced of the value of excluding refined sugar and flour products, colas, stimulants, foods processed with salt, condiments, chemical additives, etc. (We must also mention the suicidal habit of cigarette smoking here.) But as you undertake the Yoga nutrition program, your body is gradually cleansed of the influence of harmful substances, and you will experience a state of greater physical and emotional well-being. You become aware that meat can drain your vitality, that coffee can cause insomnia and irritability, that highly seasoned food can cause heartburn and indigestion, that many dairy products are responsible for mucus in the respiratory system, that sugar and sugar substitutes can adversely affect your mind and emotions, that cigarettes greatly reduce your endurance. In short, as you become sensitive to the effects of these various substances, will-power and effort are no longer necessary to curb your desire for them. More and more you are attracted to foods that provide the type of nourishment and life-force the body requires. The "wisdom of the body" makes itself felt and heard.

Rather than approach this nutrition program as an irrevocable commitment, view it as a three-month experiment. In this way, you will appease that part of you that rebels at "deprivation." Make this pact with yourself: If, at the end of a three-month period, you are not experiencing the results that have been described above, abandon the entire project and revert to your former diet, perhaps retaining certain aspects of the program that have proved their value. Ideally, during this three-month experimental period, you will dedicate yourself to the program through a diet comprised exclusively of foods high in nutritional value as described in the following pages. But if this total commitment is not possible, then a partial program can be adopted. What is true regarding *Hatha* Yoga also obtains here: You will benefit from whatever you apply, but remember that the greater your involvement, the more gratifying the results.

If you are currently under medical care, or in doubt as to the effects of the program, consult your physician before you begin.

During the past twenty-five years, several million students have applied the Yoga nutritional principles I have taught in my books, recordings, lectures, and television programs and have experienced the truth of what I have stated in this introduction. If you apply these principles, you, too, will come to understand their truth. During the three-month trial period, whatever extra effort you have to make to obtain the approved foods and to prepare them in the ways suggested in this book, will be well worthwhile.

FOOD CLASSIFICATION

FRUITS

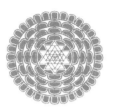

All edible fruits are good sources of energy, which is derived from their natural sugar content. In addition, they contain many nutrients and are excellent for cleansing the system. Unfortunately, many people regard fruit as little more than snacks or an occasional dessert. In our program seasonal fresh fruits constitute a major part of the daily diet. Fruits are easily and quickly digested; they are in keeping with our concept of acquiring high-quality life-force with a minimum expenditure of digestive energy.

ACID FRUITS

This category includes oranges, grapefruits, lemons, limes, tangerines, tangellos, pineapples, pomegranates, strawberries, loganberries, and cranberries. Many acid fruits are subtropical, requiring a warm, humid climate for proper growth. Oranges and grapefruits are high in vitamin C content. This essential vitamin cannot be stored in the body and must be provided on a daily basis. It is important to note that although we refer to these fruits as "acid," when consumed they have an alkaline effect. Oranges are high in fruit sugar and are a quick source of energy. Grapefruits are excellent for cleansing purposes, as is the juice of lemons and limes. Eating a breakfast of grapefruit two or three times a week can leave you feeling light and alert; your system will be cleansed and weight loss can also result. Here is a technique that has assisted those with problems of elimination: Upon arising, squeeze the juice of half a lemon into six ounces of cool water. Drink it, and after approximately fifteen minutes have elapsed, perform the Abdominal Lift exercise as instructed in the *Hatha* Yoga section.

Lemon and lime juice contain alkaline elements and citric acid, and can be used to flavor many foods, including salads. Indeed, all citrus juices are excellent and will provide varying amounts of vitamin C. These juices should be freshly squeezed and consumed shortly after squeezing. This is especially true of the orange and grapefruit.

Any citrus fruits and juices that contain sugar, preservatives, and additives are unacceptable. We advise against the use of any sweetening agent (including honey) with any fresh citrus fruit. Most people know that it is necessary to thoroughly wash the skin of fruit, but they sometimes neglect to do so with oranges, grapefruits, lemons, and limes. If these produce have been chemically sprayed, they too require washing.

Remember that many berries as well as tangerines, tangellos, pineapples, and pomegranates are also in this category and have acid fruit properties. You need not confine your selection to oranges and grapefruits.

SUBACID FRUITS

This category includes apples, apricots, peaches, plums, pears, nectarines, grapes, melons, papayas, and mangoes. Subtropical and tropical fruits such as bananas and avocados are also in this group. When fresh fruits are in season, it is often desirable to make a complete meal of fruit. In order to cleanse the system, many people eat only fresh fruits, both acid and subacid, at separate meals, for several days at a time. This is known as a fruit fast and will be explained in more detail under Fasting. You many combine as many of the subacid fruits as you wish. A meal comprised of these fruits and a nonflesh protein will leave you feeling light, satisfied, and well nourished. A popular misconception regarding bananas and avocados is that these fruits are fattening. Actually, the oils and fats in these and similar fruits are beneficial, and, if correctly combined with compatible foods and not eaten in excess, should not add extra weight. There are, of course, dozens of edible subacid fruits. We are calling attention to those that are most widely available. The juices of all subacid fruits make excellent beverages, but they must be pure, without additives or preservatives.

DRIED FRUITS

The fruits in this category include dates, figs, raisins, and currants. These provide quick energy and can be used as substitutes for refined sugar and flour products, such as cakes and candies. Children should be encouraged to eat dried fruits as snacks; they make a good lunchbox item. Other popular dried fruits are apricots, peaches, pears, and plums (prunes). All are nutritionally valuable. If necessary, you can soak dried fruits in water overnight to make them more easily digestible. A mixture of soaked fruits makes an excellent breakfast dish. Dried fruits that have been preserved with sulfur dioxide are unacceptable. Health food stores and many markets have the pure products. When free of preservatives, dried fruits are much more flavorful.

All fruits can and should, whenever possible, be eaten raw, without syrups, sweeteners, additives, preservatives, etc. If necessary, the sub-acid fruits may be baked or stewed with a small amount of honey and raisins.

Organic fruits that have not been sprayed with pesticides are our first choice. If these are unavailable, wash and scrub fruit thoroughly before eating.

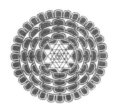

VEGETABLES

Ignorance regarding correct preparation of vegetables is widespread. They are often cooked to the point of extinction and drowned in a sauce or suffocated with condiments. All this is done in the interest of "improving the taste" of what many people consider a dull, boring part of a meal. There is a classic cartoon that appeared about forty-five years ago, showing a mother standing over a small child seated at a table with a dish of greens in front of him. The mother says. "It's broccoli, dear," and the child answers, "I say it's spinach and I say to hell with it!" But one can hardly blame the child who grows up with either a strong aversion to, or, at best, a grudging acceptance of vegetables. Why? Because too often vegetables are cooked in ways that render them tasteless (or bad-tasting) and rob them of most of their nutritional value. The greatest mistake made in the preparation of vegetables is overcooking. This is what divests them of flavor and nutritional value. When tenderized or eaten raw, they become the mainstay of our diet. Many vegetables taste better in their natural state.

FRUIT-BEARING VEGETABLES

These include tomatoes, zucchini, peppers, cucumbers, and okra. They contain varying amounts of potassium, sodium, calcium, magnesium, iron, phosphorus, and sulfur. Tomatoes, green and red peppers (good sources of vitamin C), and cucumbers can be eaten raw. These vegetables are also good for cleansing the system.

STARCH VEGETABLES

The best known of these are potatoes (all kinds), artichokes, and winter squash. The common variety of white potato is composed of water, a small amount of protein, starch, and cellulose. The sweet potato also contains sugar. Potatoes and artichokes should be baked; their starch will be used better by the body.

GREEN VEGETABLES

This category includes all varieties of lettuce, celery, chard, spinach, endive, mustard greens, parsley, cabbage, broccoli, cauliflower, brussel sprouts, and all other green leafy vegetables. These vegetables contain the most life-force and are high in nutritional value. They should be eaten in liberal quantities each day, particularly in the form of salads. If cooked, steaming is the best method. Never boil or overcook these invaluable greens; even when steamed they must remain firm. Mustard greens and cauliflower, although not usually eaten raw, should be tried this way with a natural dressing.

ROOT AND BULB VEGETABLES

Carrots, turnips, onions, beets, parsnips, radishes, garlic, rutabaga, asparagus, and horseradish are the principal vegetables in this category.

These vegetables should be cooked primarily by steaming. Raw carrots are of great nutritional value. Radishes are generally eaten raw. Most people are unaware of the value and flavor of raw turnips and asparagus tips—try them.

SPROUTS

All edible sprouts, including the mung, soy, alfafa, and bean, now frequently found in salads and sandwiches, are excellent sources of life-force. High in mineral content, they are easily digested and make satisfying snacks. You can easily learn how to grow a plentiful quantity of sprouts in your own kitchen. They can even be used as a substitute for fresh vegetables during the winter months.

MISCELLANEOUS

Fungi: mushrooms. Seaweed: kelp, dulse, carrageen. Mushrooms make an excellent main dish, as our recipes will show. Serve them raw in salads; many people find the taste of the raw mushroom much more flavorful than when cooked. Seaweed, a most nutritious item, is available in Oriental and gourmet markets.

We recommend that one meal of each day consist of a large, raw vegetable salad and/or one or more steamed or baked vegetables. If you steam vegetables, do not throw out the cooking water. Serve it as a hot drink, slightly seasoned with a vegetable salt, or as a broth, or save it as stock

for a heavier soup. This broth can be refrigerated for one day. Beyond this time it is doubtful that it retains significant value.

Whenever possible, eat the skin of the vegetable (assuming, of course, it has been thoroughly washed or scrubbed; health food stores have special kitchen items for this purpose). Many nutrients are concentrated in the skin. This is especially true of potatoes, although the skins of such vegetables as the sweet potato and the winter squash are too tough for most digestive systems. If you have access to Chinese or Japanese markets, try some of the delicious, different vegetables they carry, such as bamboo shoots, water chestnuts, and snow peas. You have probably noticed that when these vegetables are served to you in an Oriental restaurant they are always tender and crisp, never boiled and limp. You might be interested in learning the technique of stir-frying. Because vegetables are cooked quickly in this method, little nutritional value is lost.

Fresh vegetables are, of course, our first choice. Frozen vegetables are our reluctant but necessary second choice. Canned vegetables are unacceptable. Fresh vegetable juices are highly recommended as a source of easily assimilated nutrients. Juices that have been pressed or extracted with a vegetable juice machine are best. These juices can be purchased in most health food restaurants and stores; restaurants may squeeze them to order, but stores generally carry only the bottled products. When bottled they are reduced in nutritional value, but are still acceptable. A vegetable juice extractor, manufactured by a reputable firm, is a good investment in your health. Such machines are available through most larger appliance and health food stores. There are several recipes for vegetable drinks in the Recipe section of this book.

In the context of this study, the terms *organic* and *inorganic* refer primarily to the type of soil in which food is grown. "Organic" implies that the grower has prepared the soil to contain elements that will grow the most nutritious plants, bushes, trees, etc. The organic grower does not use pesticides. The manner in which your food is grown, harvested, packaged, shipped and stored should become important to you, and you should seek out the sources of organic produce in your area.

A list of suggested appliances and cooking utensils appears in the Recipe section.

PROTEINS

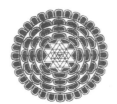

The word *protein* is of Greek derivation and means "primary" or "holding first place." This is an indication of the great importance of proteins; they are the building materials of which all living tissue is composed. You need proteins to regulate your weight, for the health of the skin, hair, and nails, and for vitality and vigor. Protein repairs and rebuilds tissues, muscles, glands, nerves, bones, and blood. Children need it to grow, and older people require it for replacing worn-out tissues.

Proteins consist of approximately 50 percent carbon, with some hydrogen, oxygen, nitrogen, traces of sulfur, and occasionally phosphorus and iron. *Amino acids* are built from these elements. There are currently twenty-three known amino acids, eight of which are considered essential. However, in Yoga nutrition, it is not enough to know that protein is necessary in the diet; we think of proteins in terms of the type and quality of life-force that they contain. Again, this life-force principle governs our selection.

In recent years the consumption of large amounts of protein, especially as a means of weight loss, has been widely advocated. We believe that excessive amounts of protein, especially in the form of powders, wafers, and animal products, not only place an unnecessary strain on the digestive system, but, in the long run, actually deplete rather than increase energy and life-force. Raising the metabolic activity of the organism through the ingestion of protein in flesh foods and concentrated protein products is not in keeping with the Yogic concept of a small, steady, controlled flow of energy. It has been our experience that in "high protein" diets whatever weight is lost is quickly regained, and whatever increase there is in vitality is lost soon after the diets are discontinued. This up-and-down pattern, continued over a long period of time, is not in the best interest of health.

In Yogic nutrition we derive our protein from such foods as cheeses, nuts, nut butters, yogurt, legumes, avocados, coconuts, mushrooms, and whole grains. This preference is based on both physiological and spiritual considerations: in addition to an aversion to mass slaughter and the belief that there can be little life-force gained from eating the body of a dead creature, flesh foods lower the vibrations of mind and spirit. The body works hard to cope with the uric acids and fibers of flesh foods, so their digestion and elimination is a chore. A meat meal leaves the body feeling heavy and the mind dulled. You can test the truth of this by abstaining from all animal products for a period of thirty days, after which you should indulge in a healthy portion of your favorite meat. The resulting lazy feeling for twenty-four hours following this meal will bring home the point in a very direct manner. The typical steer is synthetically conceived, synthet-ically fed (with waste products from various sources included in its feed mixture), and ingests doses of anti-biotics. One must seriously question how much life-force is to be derived from this creature after it is slaughtered, frozen, shipped, further dissected, "tenderized," and then cooked.

Bacon and ham are highly salted and spiced, and you have only to read the labels of these products to see that they are highly processed with chemical additives and artificial preservatives. These products as well as all smoked and pickled animal products in packages, jars, and cans, should be absolutely avoided.

Because of the quick-fattening process to which poultry is subjected (including the use of antibiotics and stilbestrol), it is, for us, little better than meat. Depending upon the waters they have inhabited and what they have eaten, fresh fish may be the least harmful of the flesh foods. Of course, it is usually very difficult to determine this, but if you know that fish comes from polluted waters, there is every reason to conclude that the fish have ingested some harmful agents, and you should avoid eating it. All fish are high in acidity. If eaten, they should have a liberal amount of lemon added; this helps to begin the digestive process, in which the acid in the fish turns to alkaline. Crustacea (shell fish such as lobster, shrimps, clams, etc.) are particularly difficult to digest.

If you wish to include some flesh foods in your diet, attempt to obtain the organic products that are available in some health food stores and markets. Flesh foods should be broiled or baked, never fried; no harsh condiments should be used in their preparation. But always be aware that progress in the objectives of Yoga will be more satisfactory if flesh foods are eliminated entirely from the diet.

EGGS

Eggs that are commercially produced for mass consumption are unfertilized, lacking in the elements to produce life. They often contain an excess of nitrogen, fat and phosphoric acid, and can be acid-forming. Fertilized eggs are preferred. Usually more flavorful and nutritious, they are available from health food stores and farms. Egg yolk is richer in iron than the albumen. If you wish to eat eggs, we recommend eating the yolk only. We consider it tragic that eggs and some form of preserved or smoked meat (ham, bacon, sausage, etc.) constitute the national breakfast. Think of what happens in the digestive system when these meats are eaten with fried or scrambled eggs, fried potatoes, toast with butter or jam, and the entire combination washed down with coffee that often contains cream and sugar! The body requires some hours to recover from such a blow and expends considerable life-force in its efforts.

Poaching or soft-boiling are the

best methods for cooking eggs. You will help to neutralize any negative effects of acid by combining eggs with the alkaline elements of vegetables and fruits. The yoke of a hard-boiled egg can be used in a green salad. A few of our recipes include eggs. If you are abstaining from all animal products, simply ignore those recipes.

The following are the proteins we recommend.

NUTS

Nuts are our primary source of plant protein. Almonds, pecans, cashews, Brazils, walnuts, and coconuts are rich in proteins, vitamins, mineral salts, sugar, starches, and oil. They are actually too rich in these substances to be thought of as a snack or something to munch on before or after meals. A few ounces of nuts can provide sufficient protein at any one meal. The fat in nuts is not to be confused with animal fats; the former is in an emulsified state that can be easily digested if not combined with incompatible foods. Nuts mix well with subacid fruits and raw vegetables. They are best consumed in an unroasted, unsalted state; they can be very lightly roasted, but never salted, and must always be thoroughly chewed. Processed nuts, which have been roasted with butter and preservatives added are not suitable for our purposes.

Nut butters are equally valuable in our program, but should be eaten either raw or very lightly roasted without additional processing. Such products are available from health food stores and some markets. Almond and cashew butters are especially good and make fine sandwiches and spreads. (The peanut is technically a legume, not a nut. However, unsalted, lightly roasted peanut butter is acceptable.)

Remember that you do not want to consume excess protein, so when nuts are included in a meal be sure to go lightly on any other proteins in that meal.

SEEDS

Sunflower, chia, pumpkin, sesame, and caraway are a few of the seeds that are recommended. A handful will provide quick energy and can be used as a snack. Again, they are best raw or very lightly roasted (not salted), and can be sprinkled on many fruit and vegetable dishes.

LEGUMES

All varieties of fresh and dried peas and beans (black-eye, lima, kidney, soy) as well as lentils and St. John's bread (carob) are popular members of this family. One serving of legumes can provide sufficient protein at a meal. In preparing legumes, it is desirable to soak them overnight. When cooking, bring the water to a boil and let simmer until tender.

The soy bean and its by-products, including the increasingly popular tofu, are exceptionally nourishing—high in protein and life-force. Soy beans are crushed to produce soy "milk," a staple food in the Orient for many centuries. St. John's bread is actually a bean; the pod is the part that is eaten and the bean is usually discarded. When it is ground it becomes carob, an excellent flavoring powder that is sweet and is now being used extensively as a healthy substitute for chocolate in pastries and candies. It can be purchased in package form and used as the base for a hot or cold beverage and for various toppings.

People who are very active and expend considerable energy will find legumes to be a particularly delicious way to satisfy their protein requirements. Because of their relatively high calorie content, however, sedentary people should consume them in moderation.

GRAINS (CEREALS, BREADS, RICE)

Whole grains are a source of protein, vitamins (especially the B complex), and minerals. Note the emphasis we place on the word *whole*. This is because most commercial flours and cereals derived from wheat, rye, barley, oats, millet, corn, and rice have been processed: quick-ground, refined, bleached, "enriched," disinfected, salted, and preserved. "Refining," in which the two most vital parts of the kernel—the embryo (wheat germ) and the bran layers—are removed, is one of the most nutritionally destructive processes that has been developed, and, we believe, is a contributing factor in malnutrition. Unfortunately, the cereals, breads, and pastries consumed by the majority of people in the Western Hemisphere are made from grains that have been subjected to this process.

Happily, whole-grain flour products are becoming increasingly popular and are now available in most markets. When you buy bread or pastry, read the label to make sure that it is made with unrefined, unbleached, and preferably stone-ground flour, and contains no preservatives or colorings. (Be careful regarding the term *whole wheat*. Most whole-wheat flour is a mixture of flours that have been processed. Remember that it is the *whole-grain* product that you want, wheat or otherwise.) Baking your own bread is a good way to ensure getting whole-grain flour.

Few whole-grain packaged cold cereals are available. Some of the "granolas" are acceptable, but, again, you must read the labels, because some have sugar and preservatives. By all means avoid those cereals that some nutritionists have labeled "sugared cardboard." These are easily identified: Read the labels and note that in addition to the processed grains and refined sugar they contain, most have the preservative BHA. You can purchase unrefined, unbleached cracked wheat, buckwheat, hominy grits, groats, cornmeal, etc. in packaged or bulk form at your health food store or market. These may be cooked, or you can make a mixture and serve them cold for breakfast. A subacid or dry fruit, milk (nonfat or raw), or yogurt can be added.

Only whole-grain (brown, wild) rice is acceptable in our program. White rice has been "polished"—a process that removes the all-important life-force germ and the layers immediately surrounding it. In addition to the ways in which rice is generally used, cooked brown rice makes an excellent breakfast food.

There are various noodle products made from a combination of grains and vegetables that can be served with a healthful sauce as the main dish of a meal. These include whole-wheat spaghetti and spinach macaroni. Some appear in our recipes. Common refined white flour pastas are not acceptable in our program.

Like legumes, grains should be eaten in moderation. Combinations of grains, such as bread and cereal, bread and rice, cereal and pastry, are not recommended.

Dairy products contain protein and are treated in the separate category that follows.

DAIRY PRODUCTS

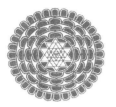

Although dairy products contain calcium, protein, and other nutrients, we advise that their consumption be carefully restricted with regard to both type and quantity. We believe that most of the elements (including calcium) of which milk is composed are better obtained from other sources and that the adverse effects of dairy products consumed in the large quantities recommended by the dairy industry far exceed their benefits.

MILK

The only milk we recommend is certified raw milk, especially nonfat, although the regular is acceptable. A farm that sells fresh milk from cows that have been inspected by the health department is an ideal source. Any dairy products made from this milk, either on the farm or by you, are acceptable. Certified raw milk can be obtained from health food stores and certain dairy companies. Some farms and health food stores carry goat's milk. We recommend goat's milk because it is more similar in composition to the milk of the human female than is cow's milk, it is more easily digested, and it is a healthier product for children.

Milk that is commercially produced is unacceptable to us. It is derived from cows that have been fed a questionable diet and have received shots of antibiotics that can be present in their milk. This milk is pasteurized (boiled) and homogenized (separated). We believe that the life-force is greatly reduced or destroyed by these processes. We contend that milk and all dairy products are highly mucus-forming and suggest that people afflicted with asthma and other respiratory ailments, including infection of the tonsils, and those suffering with arthritis should strictly limit or totally eliminate their consumption of dairy products, especially milk. It is also our contention that children, once weaned (a baby should be breast fed for at least eighteen months), require very little milk. Many pediatricians are now in accord with this view. Children who are allergic to milk, drink soy milk, derived from the soy bean.

CREAM

Certified raw cream can be purchased, but the top quarter of a bottle of raw milk will also provide cream. it should be used very sparingly. For an occasional desert you can make your own ice cream, using honey, raw cream, and natural flavoring. This is also available at health food stores and some markets, but it is always preferable to make your own. Commercial sour cream is exceptionally high in fat content and is not recommended.

YOGURT

Yogurt, acidophilus milk, and buttermilk contain cultures that aid in the digestive process. Because of its high fat content, buttermilk is not recommended. Genuine acidophilus milk is usually difficult to obtain, but if it is available at your health food store, try some. For our purposes, it is a valuable beverage.

Yogurt has been a staple food in the Balkan countries for centuries. In the past decade it has become an extremely popular item in the United States and Europe. Yogurt is made by adding bacteria cultures to fermented milk. Genuine yogurt has a tart, even sour, taste, but dairy companies, in their efforts to increase sales, have tried to make their yogurts more "palatable" by adding fruits, syrups, chocolate, and other flavorings. This is frequently the case with the popular "frozen yogurt" desserts that are promoted as "healthy" products! These commercial yogurts are unacceptable for our purposes. The best yogurt is that which you make at home. It is not hard to do and kits are available at most health food stores. The next best is natural yogurt (white, tart, without additives) available at health food stores and some markets. We question the value of yogurt that has been in a container for some days or weeks, so the fresher, the better.

Yogurt is compatible with most of the foods we have listed. It goes particularly well with fruit salads. If you eat a moderate quantity of yogurt each day, you will probably get all the dairy nutrients you require.

BUTTER

Butter made from raw milk and without salt and other additives can be very sparingly eaten. It is available at health food stores. We don't recommend regular commercial butter. Unsaturated margarines without artificial flavoring, coloring, and sodium benzoate can also be used in moderation.

CHEESE

Because most cheeses are highly processed they are unsuitable for us. They are high in fat, aged, seasoned with salt and other agents, and contain preservatives. The cheeses we recommend are uncreamed cottage cheese made with raw or nonfat milk, farmer, hoop, ricotta (Italian), feta (Greek), natural Swiss, Monterey Jack, mild cheddar, and Parmesan. The criteria for your selection should be low fat, low salt, with minimal colorings and preservatives. Cheeses can be constipating and mucus-forming so they should be combined with fruits or vegetables. They are high in protein and should be eaten in moderation, particularly at any meal in which there are other proteins.

We have included a number of recipes that call for various dairy products. If possible, try to use these products that we have described.

Beware of the products that advertise themselves as being "fortified" and "enriched." Read the labels carefully to determine which additives have been used. In our judgment, a product that requires fortification and enrichment is usually not worth eating.

SEASONINGS (SPICES, HERBS, OILS)

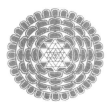

A basic objective in Yoga is learning to calm the emotions and quiet the mind. When the body is agitated, restless, or irritated, there will be a corresponding effect on the mind and emotions. In our diet, therefore, it is important to avoid those substances that will produce irritation in the digestive system, as the mind and emotions react accordingly. A person who is experiencing digestive disturbances will find it extremely difficult to quiet the mind, to meditate, and to remain generally relaxed. This is the primary reason that *Gurus* caution Yoga students against excessive use of condiments. The secondary reason is that these substances are sometimes harmful.

Therefore, we strongly urge that you eliminate the following from your diet: common table salt, all hot dog and hamburger condiments including mustard, chili, catsup, relish, pickles, and all other products that contain salt, chemical additives, and preservatives. There is no life-force in these things. They do not bring out the flavors in foods, but change, disguise, or destroy natural flavors and can cause excess acidity and heartburn. Avoid all meat, poultry, and fish sauces—both liquid and solid—commercial mayonnaise and spreads, as well as packaged and bottled salad dressings. You have only to read the label to understand why.

All "hot" condiments, including natural herbs, should be eliminated from your diet if they cause you any digestive disturbances. For example, while black pepper, chili pepper, and curry powder (consisting of ground spices) are acceptable in principle, they may affect you adversely. Decide for yourself which you can tolerate.

We urge Yoga students to minimize their consumption of foods containing common table salt. Used by processors, packagers, and shippers as a preservative because it retards decay and thereby prolongs shelf life, salt dries, hardens, constricts, ossifies, and tightens. It is an inorganic substance; its harmful effects are now becoming widely known. More and more physicians are prescribing salt-free diets to combat certain illnesses. Organic salts required by the body can be derived from the foods we have discussed in this section.

Almost all seasonings increase thirst, causing one to drink more fluids than necessary. We believe that there is no value in increased consumption of fluids that places an added burden on the stomach and kidneys. So we advise moderation in condiments, even when in their natural state. As you begin to eat more natural foods and eliminate processed foods, your taste buds will regain their original sharpness, and you will find that you require less and less seasoning for enjoyment of your food.

Here are a few of the seasonings that can be used sparingly in the Yoga program: mild herbs (basil and thyme, for example, are mild in comparison with pepper and mustard), fresh garlic, onions, parsley, lemon juice, soy bean derivatives, (tamari, for example) pure cider vinegar. If you must use salt, use sea salt or a vegetable salt substitute. There are dozens of natural condiments. You may use whichever you feel conform to the above-stated principles.

We suggest using cold-pressed, unrefined, nonanimal oils for seasonings and cooking. These include safflower, olive, and sesame oil; they are available from health food stores and some markets.

SUGAR

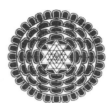

If we were to select the single substance that is the most harmful staple in the Western diet, it would have to be refined white sugar. It is almost impossible to find a packaged, canned, or bottled food in the supermarket to which salt, or sugar, or both have not been added. Yet the elimination of these "deadly twins" for the diet would vastly improve the general health of the entire population.

Again, the process of "refinement" enters the picture. Here, part of the process involves extracting the sugar from the cane or beet, thus separating it from essential elements required for its healthful digestion. Divested of these elements, sugar cannot be properly assimilated. In excess, sugar can contribute to obesity, cause irritability, and depression. It depletes the B vitamins, draws calcium from the gums, and changes the mineral relationships in the body. The quick energy that results from consuming a candy bar or cola is due to the sudden rise of the blood sugar level, but the level drops as quickly as it rose, and then more sugar is required to compensate for this sudden depletion. In this way one becomes a sugar "addict." Its negative effects have been the subject of entire books, but the characteristic of refined sugar that is the most important to remember for purposes of Yoga nutrition is this: More surely and quickly than any other substance, sugar destroys life-force.

The various chemical substitutes

for sugar that are used in diet foods, beverages, chewing gum, etc. and promoted as being valuable because they are "sugar free" and "low calorie" are to be strictly avoided. Fortunately, the federal government has banned the use of certain cyclamates, although certain special-interest groups are working to have this ban rescinded. We consider these chemical substitutes to be even more harmful than refined sugar.

Here are the sources of sugar we recommend, in order of preference based on nutritional value: Fresh fruits, dried fruits, molasses (rich in iron), pure maple syrup and sugar, beet sugar (derived from eating beets that have not been overcooked), cane sugar (from chewing cane stalk), carob (chew the pod of the bean or use the powder), honey (unbleached and uncooked; it's a highly concentrated food and should be consumed very sparingly), raw sugar, and brown sugar. With these alternatives, there is no reason to include refined white sugar in your diet for even another day.

Based on our views regarding homogenized, pasteurized milk and sugar, syrups, and chemical sweetening agents, you will readily understand our aversion to colas, ice cream beverages, "punches," and all frozen, concentrated, canned, and bottled drinks that contain these substances.

BEVERAGES

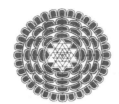

Beverages that negatively affect the nervous system should also be eliminated from the diet. Depression, irritability, restlessness, insomnia, and damage to the digestive system and brain can result from alcohol, the caffeine in coffee, and the caffeine, bromide, and tannic acid in many commercial teas. From our point of view, a person who drinks several cups of coffee each day and/or indulges in several cocktails is flirting with as much danger as a chain-smoker. Caffeine is an addicting drug and is probably a contributing factor in certain mental and emotional disorders. Many people experience relief of the symptons of nervous disorders by simply eliminating coffee and sugar from their diets. Commercial teas containing tannic acid are not much better than coffee, although a cup of tea contains slightly less caffeine than coffee.

The harmful physical effects of alcohol are universally known. We believe that people who insist that it is "safe in moderate amounts" are fooling themselves. It has an adverse, cumulative effect on the stomach and liver in any amount. From the Yogic viewpoint, an ever greater danger lies in the fact that the ingestion of a substance that artificially alters the consciousness will weaken the mind and willpower and thus seriously retard progress in the practice of Yoga. This is also true of such substances as marijuana, "uppers" and "downers," heroin, cocaine, hashish, LSD, etc. Once the initial sensation of relaxation and/or exhilaration has worn off, the body is left inert and the mind dulled. One cannot be seriously engaged in Yogic practice while these consciousness-altering agents are used. If you currently take caffeine, alcohol, or any other mind-altering substances, your Yoga program of exercises, nutrition, and meditation will produce a consistent, natural elation that will reduce your desire for artificial stimulants.If you must include alcohol in your diet, the least harmful are light white and red wines.

One of the primary substances of life-force is water. It is therefore of great importance that it is *pure*. For us, "pure" means fresh and uncontaminated by pollutants and chemicals. Water that contains fluoride, for example, is not acceptable; we prefer to prevent tooth decay through proper nutrition that includes the elimination of tooth-decaying foods. If you do not have access to your own source of pure water, certain bottled waters will serve the purpose. These are delivered by bottled water distributors and are also available in markets. We emphasize that *only pure water as defined above should be used for drinking and in cooking.*

All freshly squeezed or extracted fruit and vegetable juices are high in nutritional value and life-force. Bottled products available in health food stores and some markets are acceptable, but, of course, some nutritional value is lost as these products "age" on store shelves.

A great variety of herb teas containing many healthful properties are available. These and cereal beverages (made from a mixture of grains) should be used in place of coffee, tea, and chocolate. Do not resort to "low-caffeine" products; eliminate caffeine entirely. Powdered chocolate and tea beverages are equally unacceptable. Read the labels and you will see why.

Vegetable broths that are derived from the steaming of your vegetables are nourishing and can be drunk as teas. Vegetable bouillon cubes and powders without chemicals, additives, and preservatives are acceptable.

We advise against drinking any beverage during or immediately following a meal, because liquid interferes with the digestive process. In general, beverages consumed should be cool or warm not extremely hot or ice cold.

FOOD SUPPLEMENTS

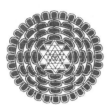

We believe that a diet containing an abundance of fruits and vegetables, proteins in moderation, and, if desired, dairy products—all from the sources suggested in these pages—will seldom require supplementation. If, however, your diet is inadequate in fresh fruits, raw vegetables, natural proteins, and fats, one or more supplements may be advisable. Wheat germ, brewer's yeast, natural gelatin, rice polishings, and rose hips are just a few of the many supplements that are available. (A number of these are used in our recipes.) Always exercise prudence in your use of these supplements. They can be expensive and fill the body with more of certain substances than it requires. This overabundance can create as many problems as any deficiency can.

SUMMARY

RECOMMENDED

Fresh or bottled spring water.

Freshly squeezed fruit and vegetable juices. Bottled and frozen products without additives are acceptable, but much lower in life-force.

Herb teas and cereal beverages.

Vegetable broths and bouillons (without common salt).

Raw nonfat milk, and products made from this milk, including cheese, butter, yogurt, custard, and ice cream.

Goat's milk.

Acidophilus milk (must be pure, not mixed with other types of milk).

Fertilized eggs (very sparingly).

Whole grain products, including baked items, cereals, brown rice, and pastas.

All edible fresh fruits and vegetables. If fresh product is unavailable, frozen items are acceptable.

Legumes: dried peas, lentils, beans such as lima, pinto, soy; soy bean products.

Soups, see the recipes.

Nuts, as specified under Proteins.

Nut butters.

Seeds: sunflower, pumpkin, etc.

Dried fruits.

Cheese, as specified under Proteins.

Seasonings: mild herbs, vegetable salt, polyunsaturated oils.

Margarine, unsaturated.

Sweeteners: molasses, honey, carob, pure maple syrup and maple sugar, raw sugar.

NOT RECOMMENDED

Water to which chemicals, including fluoride, have been added.

Homogenized, pasteurized milk and products made from this milk, including buttermilk, sour cream, cheese, butter, ice cream.

Coffee, tea, and all products containing caffeine.

All bottled, frozen, concentrated, and canned fruits and fruit juices, and vegetables and vegetable juices containing additives and preservatives (salt, sugar, syrup, etc.).

Yogurts flavored with fruits and syrups.

Unfertilized eggs.

Alcoholic beverages.

Common salt and all products containing this salt (which includes many cheeses).

Strong spices and condiments, and the seasonings, sauces, dressings, spreads, cheeses, and other preparations made from them, most of which contain chemical additives and preservatives.

Smoked, marinated, and pickled products.

Refined grain products, including breads, crackers, muffins, pies, cakes, cookies, white rice, cereals, and pastas.

Meat, poultry, and fish. This includes ham, bacon, salami, pastrami, "luncheon" meats, and all products containing animal substances.

Refined sugar and products that contain refined sugar: pastries, puddings, candies, jellies, jams, chewing gum, ice cream, colas, syrups.

Chemical sugar substitutes. These are usually promoted as "low calorie" and found in colas, confections, and many "diet foods."

"Instant" breakfasts, appetite deterrents, and "high protein" products. Wafers, powders, tablets, breads, cereals, candies, and beverages are popular forms for these products.

Foods that have been prepared by frying, boiling, pressure-cooking, in microwave ovens, in animal fats, or that simply appear "greasy."

The overriding principle is to be wary of all foods and beverages that have been sprayed, aged, colored, emulsified, thickened, boiled, fried, smoked, marinated, bleached, refined and otherwise processed, and that contain preservatives. The labels usually tell enough of the story for you to make a decision. We do not attempt to disguise the fact that strict application of this principle will eliminate 98 percent of the foods that comprise the average diet.

MENUS

These menus will serve as examples of the foods that are used in the program. An infinite number of combinations are possible for each meal. All of the foods and beverages are detailed in the pertinent categories, and the recipe for each dish can be found in the recipe section. A beverage of your choice (herb tea, etc.) can be included with any meal, but we suggest that this be taken a short time following the meal.

BREAKFAST

Half grapefruit

1/2 cup nuts (of your choice)

Dish of berries in season

Date-nut shake (p.112)

Dish of sliced fresh peaches, figs, and bananas

Baked apple with honey and raisins

Whole grain toast with fruit butter

Dish of fried prunes (soaked overnight in water and lemon juice)

Steamed brown rice with honey and cinnamon

LUNCH

Zucchini Pancakes with yogurt-herb sauce (p.142)

Tomato slices with herb dressing

Carob macaroons (p.162)

Avocado, grapefruit, and cottage cheese salad

Whole grain crackers

Quesadilla (p.110)

Gazpacho (p.118)

Grapes

Lentil soup (p.116)

Whole grain crackers

Spinach salad with lemon juice dressing

DINNER

Wild rice and mushrooms (p.136)

Green salad with tomato-basil dressing

Banana-orange sherbet (p.159)

Nut loaf with tamari gravy (p.145)

Green bean salad (p.123)

Applesauce cake (p.160)

Spinach quiche (p.139)

Greek salad (p.124)

Fresh fruit compote with yogurt topping

Yogurt soup (p.116)

Vegetable curry with lemon rice (p.132)

Pineapple spears

BREAKFAST	LUNCH	DINNER
Orange juice Cold grain cereal with raw milk and sliced banana	Avocado sandwich with alfalfa sprouts on whole grain bread Fresh fruit	Ratatouille (p.137) Romaine Salad with French dressing Baked pears
Raw applesauce with yogurt Whole grain toast with margarine or fruit butter	Fresh tomato scooped out and filled with herb garden cottage cheese Sesame wheat crackers (p.108) Fresh, crisp apple	Sprouted wheat burgers with cashew gravy (p.145) Bean sprout salad Fruit juice gelatin
Fresh grapefruit juice Buckwheat pancakes (p.152) with pure maple syrup, honey, or molasses	Fruit butter and cream cheese sandwich on whole grain raisin bread Fresh fruit	Rice stuffed peppers (p.135) Raw vegetable sticks dipped in guacamole (p.125) Honey carrot ice cream (p.159)
Grape-apple blender drink Wheat germ muffins (p.148) with margarine or fruit butter	Mushroom-cheese sandwich Green salad with Tahini dressing (p.130)	Corn chowder (p.121) Artichoke with yogurt-herb sauce Crispy topped apples (p.153)

BREAKFAST	LUNCH	DINNER
Cantaloupe	Fresh carrot juice	Filled cabbage leaves (p.139)
Thermos bottle—cooked cereal topped with chopped dates and cinnamon	Dried fruit salad	Raw pea salad (p.123)
	Zucchini cupcake with cream cheese frosting (p.162)	Eggless rice pudding (p.158)
Carob-honey blender shake (p.112)	Fresh apple juice	Egg foo yung (p.134)
Dish of dried apricots, dates, and almonds	Sesame crackers with nut butter and honey	Mixed green salad with thousand island dressing
	Carrot sticks	Papaya-pineapple dessert (p.127)

LUNCHBOX SUGGESTIONS

Sandwiches (on whole grain bread)

Mushroom-cheese

Avocado and sprouts

Cashew butter with honey

Cream cheese on banana bread

Miscellaneous

Apricot leather

Nuts and dried fruits

Raw vegetable sticks

Mineral-rich potato curls

Fresh fruits (apples, peaches, etc.)

In a nonplastic container with tight lid

Ratatouille (p.137)

Kidney, garbanzo, and string bean salad; carrot-raisin salad

Herb garden cottage cheese

Fruit compote (p.153,154)

Blender applesauce

Yogurt with fruit slices

Thermos bottle

Most drinks listed under Beverages

SOURCES OF RECOMMENDED FOODS

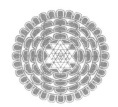

If there is any possibility of growing your own vegetables and fruits, you should seriously consider it. Even a small plot of land can yield a surprising supply of produce. All efforts you may have to make to overcome the obstacles that prevent you from becoming your own grower will be very worthwhile. The satisfaction of having fresh, organic produce cannot be surpassed, in terms of both taste and nourishment. If you are now growing your own foods, you are well aware of the truth of this statement.

Barring the possibility of your growing or otherwise producing your own foods, attempt to locate a farm that sells organic produce and/or the raw milk products that have been recommended. It is usually necessary to seek out several farms in order to obtain a variety of vegetables, fruits, dairy products, and nuts.

Some markets have the recommended products. Again, it is usually necessary to patronize a number of markets and outlets to obtain foods of the various categories. One market will have natural grain products; you may find a roadside stand that sells organic vegetables and freshly squeezed fruit and/or vegetable juices; there are bakery outlets that have bread and pastry without additives and preservatives; certain dairy companies deliver raw milk, butter, cheese, and yogurt; some farmers markets have organic fruits, nuts, and fertilized eggs. Make inquiries, and the necessary sources will begin to materialize.

Probably the best source for obtaining the widest variety of the recommended items is a large health food store. Under one roof you will find the whole grain products, raw milk products, fertilized eggs, unprocessed nuts, herb teas, cereal beverages, pure fruit and vegetable juices, and possibly organic produce. When you become familiar with several of the health food stores in your community, you may find that the quality of the recommended items varies among them; this is particularly true of the produce. Make your selections at each store accordingly. People who work in health food stores that do not carry organic produce often know where it can be obtained. A telephone call to a health food restaurant can also turn up a good source of produce.

If you live in an area where many of the recommended items are difficult to obtain, simply do the best you can.

WEIGHT REGULATION

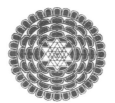

The Yoga exercises in Part I are designed to help stimulate and promote the correct functioning of organs and glands that help to regulate and correctly distribute weight, and that receive so little conscious attention in sports and the various systems of calisthenics. We have previously indicated that the complete *Hatha* Yoga program will assist you in regulating, redistributing, and controlling your weight. In addition, you can emphasize various areas of your body for these purposes by following the suggestions under Weight Control in the Yoga for Problems section.

The Yoga nutrition program will also be of great assistance to you in regulating and controlling your weight. Each person who is overweight has an *individual* problem; metabolisms and many other critical factors vary. The amount of food that constitutes overeating, or the kind of food from which excess calories are derived, can be much different for you than for a friend or other members of your family. Therefore, it becomes extremely important for you to become sensitive to *your* body, to listen to what it is telling you in regard to the weight at which it best functions and how the foods and combination of foods in your diet affect it. This type of sensitivity implies more and more self-reliance; you cannot learn such things from other people and literature that want to tell you about *your* health and well-being. Calorie charts, weight tables, and "miracle" diets are of no interest to those who have become attuned to the real requirements of their bodies.

These self-examination and self-reliance principles are to be applied in our nutrition program. First, you must have a clear and realistic concept of what your correct weight should be. If, for example, you are a large-boned woman, you cannot model your measurements after the mannequins of the fashion magazines or TV commercials. Pursuing this fantasy will not only frustrate you, but can result in serious physical harm. A small-boned man with a slight skeleton will experience the same difficulties if he is determined to acquire the appearance of a linebacker. Increased metabolic activity results from deliberately setting the body on fire with large quantities of meats, poultry, fish, eggs, powders, wafers, and other "high protein" products. Appetite deterrents designed to reduce the normal desire for nourishment, a forced cigarette and coffee diet, the synthetic products that are consumed in liquid form as a substitute for food, and most of the "miracle" diets that contain the "low calorie" sugar substitutes and other horrendous additives are in conflict with our concept of natural, healthful and permanent weight regulation. These things *oppose*, rather than assist the way in which your body wants to function; they never feel comfortable because they are unnatural, and so you have a sense of being permanently at war with yourself.

For most people who give it a fair trial, the Yoga way of eating becomes permanent. They have no desire to deviate from this diet, and if they do deviate they return to it—usually without much delay—because the negative results from the deviation are immediate and pronounced. Having a few such experiences will be more convincing than all the words we can write on the subject. The point is that we are able to assist our permanent weight regulation through a natural, life-force diet, and we remain on this diet because it is the one with which we feel our best, physically, emotionally, and mentally.

Because of the above-mentioned *individuality* of each person, we offer no specific diets or menus in this book for those who have a weight problem. If you have such a problem, simply apply the principles and follow the suggestions of the program as it is presented in this section. But if you are overweight, a period of fasting should be regularly undertaken (see Fasting), and you must carefully restrict your intake of dairy products, sweeteners, and the natural fats contained in nuts, nut butters, avocados, oil, and whatever other substances you sense may add excess weight. Watch and listen to your body and it will inform you of what these substances are. Remember that as you increase your life-force, you will become acutely aware of the body's requirements. A powerful, unmistakable instinct directs you to those foods and activities that will be beneficial and away from those that will prove harmful.

In undertaking the Yoga posture and nutrition program for assisting you with a weight problem (or any problem), *be patient.* A physical condition that has taken some years to manifest cannot be eliminated overnight. Although in certain situations students have experienced dramatic improvements within a brief period of time, it is the general rule that nature works in a methodical and progressive manner. Rather than anticipating instantaneous miracles, recognize that with Yoga you are engaged in the very finest natural program to *assist* nature in accomplishing, according to its own plan, what is necessary. Results that are achieved through the steady and patient application of Yoga will be far more rewarding and have a much better chance of becoming permanent than those that may be experienced through the devices and gimmicks used in an attempt to shortcut nature's way.

FAMILY, SOCIAL, AND RESTAURANT DINING

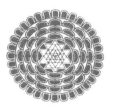

The large majority of our students are practicing Yoga within the context of family, business, and social life. The nutrition program must become a part of that life. This frequently requires modifications in one's daily habits and patterns. But once they understand the great value of these changes, students find the ways to make the necessary adjustments.

For example, a woman who is a wife and mother—concerned about and largely responsible for the health of her family—and who becomes interested in Yoga nutrition, inevitably comes to understand the importance of having her family's diet conform with its principles. In many cases the members of the family will also understand the value of eating this way, once the theory is explained to them and they taste the various wholesome, nutritious dishes that can be prepared. Experiencing an improvement in health, or simply a feeling of lightness and well-being, they come to see that eliminating or strictly limiting their consumption of animal products, processed, and denatured foods is in their best interests. In these cases, there are few problems for the homemaker. But if members of families do not so readily adapt to such modifications, the wife/mother must cope with the situation as best she can. It may be necessary for her to prepare one type of meal for herself and another for her husband and children. But with patience and ingenuity she will be able to devise many ways in which to introduce the more wholesome foods into the family's diet and reduce sugar, refined flour, and animal products. No specific instructions can be given, but many of the substitutions suggested in this section could be made immediately without causing conflict. It is an interesting fact that more and more knowledgable youngsters are attempting to convert their parents to a diet of unprocessed food.

Mothers with babies will find that with the use of a blender an infinite number of natural food preparations can be devised. Many of the commercial "baby foods" are denatured, cooked, and processed, and contain additives and preservatives. Reading the labels will cause any intelligent mother to think twice before feeding her baby these foods.

Dining at another person's home, or at a restaurant, is also a situation in which you must make the best of the circumstances. If, without going into details, you let it be known that you are simply "on a diet," you can often pass up those dishes that you definitely do not want to eat, and not offend the host by doing so. It is best not to discuss your Yoga nutrition program with those who are not totally sympathetic because you will find yourself in the position of having to either defend the program, or convince others of its value. It has been our experience that much life-force is expended in such discussions and, usually, nothing is accomplished. In the beginning, the less you speak about your Yoga diet, the better. Eventually, you will know when the time is right for you to advise another person regarding his or her diet and you will then be able to offer this advice in a gentle and knowledgeable manner.

In most restaurants you can order fruit, salad, a vegetable plate, etc. There are now numerous restaurants that are wholly dedicated to the serving of natural foods. These are being frequented for lunch and dinner by an ever increasing number of health-minded people. Depending upon the extent of the menu, you may have anything from a sandwich and herb tea to a full-course family dinner. Dining at a natural food gourmet restaurant can be a delightful experience; you will encounter delicious combinations of fruits, vegetables, and grains and these will inspire you in your own food preparation.

Vegetable dinners at Japanese and Chinese restaurants can be acceptable, depending upon the type of cooking and seasonings that are used. Most oriental chefs are inclined to use stronger and greater quantities of seasonings than we have recommended. Also, many of the dishes are prepared by frying. But there are exceptions; you must use your judgment.

The most important thing to remember in refusing any food offered or served to you in another person's home or in a restaurant is to be gracious and inoffensive so that no ill feelings are generated.

FASTING

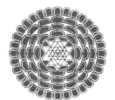

Fasting is a technique used since time immemorial to achieve physical and spiritual objectives. Because of its effectiveness and the fact that it is utilized by the Yogi, fasting is included in this section as an aspect of serious Yoga practice.

Fasting is not to be confused with starving. Fasting is the voluntary abstention from food. In Yoga, the fast is undertaken primarily to cleanse and renew, as part of a program of regeneration. When the digestive system is permitted to rest through abstention from food, a cleansing process is initiated; this process continues as long as the fast is in effect. A person who understands its purpose, and is psychologically prepared, can fast for many weeks. This is done by thousands of people. In fasting sanitariums, a fast of two to three months is not unusual. Lengthy fasts are possible because at any given time there are considerable amounts of food substances stored in the body; indeed, the problem for most people is that there is far too much food stored! Certain symptoms signal the point at which a fast should be terminated. Unless food is ingested at that point, the body will feed upon itself. This marks the end of fasting and the beginning of starvation.

Lengthy fasting is, of course, undertaken only under special circumstances that include supervision by an authority. The fast that is practical for the person in the average living situation is what we will refer to as a "partial" fast. This may take three forms. In the first, you select a day during which you can rest and relax; on that day you eat nothing at all; you drink pure water only when thirsty. Most people find this total rest for the body and digestive system a welcome relief; some experience a minor headache or irritability, which results from the cleansing process that is quickly initiated. This is especially true of those who are exceptionally toxic from coffee, meat, and refined sugar. If you remain as quiet as possible, the negative symptoms will be minimized. Attempt to avoid any contact with the sight or odor of food. The following morning, you resume eating with a very light breakfast or only a glass of fresh juice. You then continue your meals according to the program. After several of these one-day-per-week fasts, you can undertake a two-to-three-day fast when circumstances permit. The ideal plan would then be to fast one day per week and extend the fast to two or three days once each month. The Yogi feels that this type of weekly fasting has many benefits: it is cleansing, assists in weight regulation, and helps to renew the organism. The fast should not be extended beyond three days without competent supervision.

The second form of the partial fast is the elimination of one or two meals for several consecutive days. Breakfast is the logical meal to eliminate; many Yoga students find that they function more efficiently and feel more energetic by permanently eliminating breakfast. Lunch can be skipped if you are not in a working situation that day. You would implement this plan on one or more days of each week. This form of the partial fast is considerably more moderate than the previous one, but can be very helpful for those who wish to reduce the number of their meals and find that total abstention for one or more days is too difficult. The theory here is simple: Periodic elimination of a meal is more beneficial than having that meal. Of course, these plans are always carried out in conjunction with the Yoga nutrition program.

The third form of the partial fast is the eating of only one type of food at all meals for a comfortable period of time. Fresh fruits in season, particularly the watermelon, grape, peach, apricot, pear, and papaya, are best for this purpose. A more intensive form of this plan is to limit yourself to freshly squeezed fruit and vegetable juices for several consecutive days. If you experiment intelligently, you will soon work out a plan of fasting that is of the most value for your needs. It is not mandatory to fast in order to succeed with your Yoga program, but this is a technique that has been extremely beneficial to many students and deserves your consideration.

Fasting is an instinctive method of coping with an illness, and you should be aware of it in this context. When an animal becomes ill, you cannot make it eat. It knows that its recuperative power is impaired by eating, so it will find a quiet place, lie down, and not take nourishment until it is well. Man also frequently loses his appetite during an illness. His body wants to use its life-force to repair and heal, not to digest additional substances that it doesn't require. But unheeding, and believing it is necessary to "keep up his strength," he force-feeds himself, thereby complicating the condition and extending its duration. It is another situation in which the wisdom of the body is disregarded. To us, the onset of an illness usually signals that the body has been abused and that what is required are rest and *fasting*. Knowing this can be of great value to you.

In all religious scriptures there are references to "fasting." Many people think that fasting in its spiritual context is punitive, that is denotes denial, deprivation, or self-imposed punishment as a form of repentance. This is not the case, and is particularly inaccurate from the Yogic viewpoint. During the fast, there is an elation and spirituality that is difficult to explain; it must be experienced to be understood. When abstaining from food, the physical aspect of existence becomes less of a reality and the spiritual aspect—the knowledge that you are not the body—emerges. This is an exhilarating, joyous experience. If you fast regularly and meditate during these fasts, you will become aware of why the great saints and spiritual leaders in every part of the world have, throughout history, fasted to gain inspiration, strength, and spiritual insight.

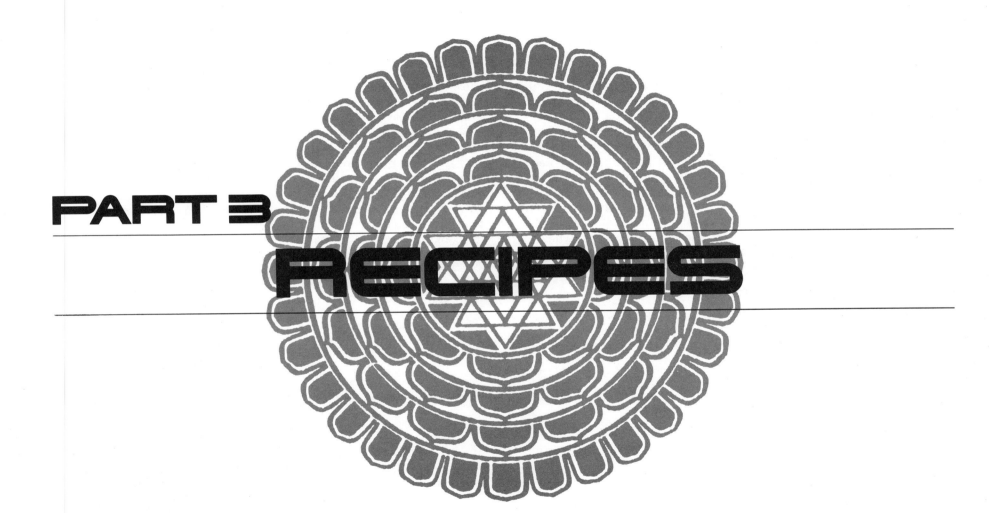

PART 3
RECIPES

RECIPE NOTES

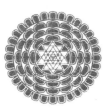

All foods used in the recipes should be the kinds recommended in Part II. For example, "milk" means raw milk; "yogurt" means unadulterated commercial yogurt or homemade yogurt; "salt" means vegetable or sea salt; "eggs" means fertilized eggs; "water" means pure water, etc. If you are in doubt about the recommended foods, refer to the pertinent categories in Part II.

Some items with which you may be unfamiliar are usually found in health food stores and certain markets—powdered kelp, herb teas, brewer's yeast, wheat-germ powder, rice polish, sesame protein powder (not to be confused with the "high-protein weight loss" products, which we do not recommend), sunflower meal, carob powder, whole-wheat pastry flour, etc. (See "Sources of the Recommended Foods" in Part II.)

Instructions for making yogurt, tofu, nut butters, tahini, and fruit butters, and for sprouting are included among the recipes. Unless otherwise indicated, "flour" means whole-wheat flour, whole grain. "Pastry flour" means whole-wheat pastry flour, which is of a finer grind. "Baking powder" should be of a low-sodium content; Royal is one brand that meets this requirement. A few of the pastry recipes call for a very small quantity of baking soda. Arrowroot is a nutritious starch containing an alkaline ash with calcium content. It is derived from the rootstocks of the arrowroot plant. It is used as a thickening agent instead of cornstarch.

The cooking direction "sauté" is not to be confused with frying. When we sauté, we cook in an uncovered pan with unsaturated oil or margarine, stirring only until tender.

If fresh fruits and vegetables are unavailable, frozen products may be used. There are many recipes calling for fruits, vegetables, nuts, and condiments in which substitutions may be made according to availability. Do not be reluctant to experiment with substitutions, particularly in a situation where you can substitute a fresh item for one that is frozen or canned. If a recipe contains a food that you do not wish to eat, either substitute another ingredient or simply disregard that recipe.

Main dish recipes make approximately five servings unless otherwise indicated.

SUGGESTED APPLIANCES AND UTENSILS

Blender or food processor*

Electric mixer

Citrus juicer

Juice extractor

Yogurt incubator

Food grinder

Nut mill

Shredder and grater

Heat-resistant casseroles, glass or stoneware

Enamel-coated cast iron pans with tight-fitting lids

Stainless steel saucepans with tight-fitting lids

Soup kettle

Loaf, pie, and cake pans

Metal burner pad

Unless made with high-grade, heavy-gauge aluminum, we advise against the use of aluminum utensils. Because of the softness of the compound, lower grades of aluminum can interact with foods.

Until irrefutable proof as to the radiation safety of microwave ovens has been offered, we strongly advise against their use. Even if such proof is forthcoming it would not change our opposition to the type of molecular alteration that occurs in food subjected to accelerated cooking.

A food processor, fitted with the steel blade, may be used in all the recipes in this section that call for the use of a blender. And, of course, you may want to use a food processor to chop, slice, shred, etc. Follow the instructions of the manufacturer.

HOMEMADE YOGURT

1 quart nonfat raw milk
½ to 1 cup nonfat dry milk powder
¼ cup yogurt

1. Combine raw milk with milk powder in 2-quart saucepan and mix well. Place over low heat until mixture reaches 180°F (82°C), stirring constantly. Cover and let cool to 110°F (43°C).

2. Add yogurt. Stir with wire whisk until mixed. Strain mixture into clean 5-cup container. Incubate at 100°F to 110°F (38°C to 43°C) until thick, 3 to 10 hours (time will vary with temperature and type of yogurt used). Cover and refrigerate.

Places that may stay 100°F (38°C):

1. Top of hot water heater. Wrap container in thick towel.

2. Gas oven with pilot light. Wrap container in thick towel.

3. Large pot with cover and 2 inches of 115°F (46°C) water in bottom, placed over pilot light on stove. For additional heat, wrap covered pot in thick towels.

4. Commercial yogurt maker.

Makes 1 generous quart.

APPETIZERS, SPREADS, SANDWICHES

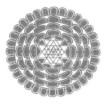

SESAME WHEAT CRACKERS

1 cup whole-wheat flour
¼ cup oil
¼ teaspoon sea salt
2 teaspoons (about) cold water
Sesame seeds

1. Combine flour, oil, and salt in medium bowl and blend with fork until mixture resembles coarse meal. Add water and mix lightly, just until dough holds together; do not over-mix. Chill several hours or overnight.

2. Preheat oven to 350°F (175°C). Lightly oil baking sheet. Roll dough out very thin on lightly floured surface. Cut with knife, pastry wheel, or cookie cutter. Arrange on prepared baking sheet. Sprinkle with sesame seeds. Bake until crisp and golden, about 10 minutes.

Makes about 2 dozen.

HORS D'OEUVRES

A tray of varied cheeses is always tantalizing party fare. Such a tray might include:

Natural Cheddar
Natural Swiss
Monterey Jack
Sweet Muenster
Feta

A pleasant complement to a cheese tray is a platter of fresh fruit, such as:

Apples
Papayas
Pineapple spears
Stuffed prunes
Peaches

It's always best to make your own crackers, but many whole-grain crackers without preservatives are available. The sesame seed variety is especially good. Pumpernickel, rye, and most whole-grain breads are attractive sliced very thin, with each slice cut into quarters or thirds. Each piece can be topped with a filling or spread, such as:

Cheddar cheese and grated apple
Avocado, chives, and lemon juice
Cream cheese and alfalfa sprouts
Artichoke hearts with olive oil and lemon
Cheddar cheese topped with black olive
Nut butter

NUT BUTTER

1 to 2 tablespoons sesame or soy oil
1 cup raw nuts. Choose from cashews, almonds, walnuts, filberts, pignolias, Brazil nuts. (The peanut is a legume, but can be used.)

1. Combine nuts and oil in blender or food processor fitted with steel blade and blend at high speed until mixture becomes a thick paste.

2. Some nuts, such as cashews, will need little or no oil; experiment.

Makes about 1 cup.

MINERAL-RICH POTATO PEEL CURLS

Potatoes
Margarine or oil

1. Scrub raw potatoes with stiff brush under running water. Cut off thick slices of peeling.

2. Heat margarine or oil in heavy large skillet over medium-high heat. Add potato peelings and sauté until curled and cooked through. Serve immediately.

Note: leftover potato centers are excellent dough conditioners for bread making. Just boil and puree in blender with the water they were cooked in; use in place of plain water. Potato water improves the flavor of all baked goods.

GARBANZO-SESAME SPREAD

¾ cup uncooked garbanzo beans,
   or 2 cups, cooked
1 pound tahini (sesame seed butter,
   available in most health food
   stores. If unavailable, grind ¾ cup
   sesame seeds in blender, a small
   amount at a time. To this meal,
   add enough sesame oil to make a
   thick paste.)
¼ cup olive oil
2 tablespoons finely chopped green
   onion
2 tablespoons chopped parsley
2 teaspoons sea salt

1. To cook beans, soak overnight in
water to cover. Rinse, cover with
water, and cook over medium heat
until soft enough to mash, about 2
hours.

2. Mash cooked garbanzo beans.

3. Add tahini and blend well.

4. Stir in remaining ingredients and
chill thoroughly. Excellent on whole-
grain bread, topped with alfalfa
sprouts.

Makes about 3 cups.

FRUIT BUTTER

7 to 8 apples, peeled, cored and
   sliced (other fruits may be used,
   including peaches, apricots,
   plums, nectarines)
½ cup honey
Cinnamon, to taste
Cloves, to taste
Ginger, to taste
Mace, to taste

Combine apples, honey, and spices
in large saucepan. Add enough water
to cover. Bring to boil over high heat.
Reduce heat and simmer until reduced to thick brown paste, about 3
to 4 hours, stirring occasionally. Puree
in blender or food processor if a
smoother consistency is desired.

Makes about 6 cups.

HOMEMADE CREAM CHEESE

1. Let 1 quart fresh raw whipping
cream stand at room temperature
until it sours, about 24 hours.

2. Pour soured cream into clean
cheesecloth bag. Suspend over bowl
to catch dripping whey. Let drain
completely, several hours or
overnight.

3. Mold cheese into 2 small cakes.
Wrap tightly and refrigerate.

Makes about ½ pound.

TOFU SALAD SANDWICH SPREAD

½ pound tofu
3 tablespoons chopped celery
2 tablespoons chopped green onion
1 tablespoon homemade mayonnaise
½ teaspoon chopped parsley
½ teaspoon celery seeds
¼ teaspoon dill weed
¼ teaspoon turmeric
¼ teaspoon vegetable salt

Crumble tofu into medium bowl.
Blend in all remaining ingredients.
Especially good on toasted whole-
grain rye bread.

Makes about 1 cup.

CREAM CHEESE WITH CHIVES

3 ounces cream cheese, preferably
   homemade
¼ cup chopped black olives
1 tablespoon chives or green onion,
   chopped

Blend all ingredients. Cover and
refrigerate.

Makes about ½ cup.

MUSHROOM-CHEESE SANDWICH FILLING

2 tablespoons oil
½ cup chopped mushrooms
¼ cup chopped onion
½ cup grated Monterey Jack cheese
½ cup grated cheddar cheese
½ cup chopped spinach leaves
¼ cup sunflower seeds
¼ cup grated carrot
¼ cup yogurt or homemade
    mayonnaise

Heat oil in medium skillet over medium heat. Add mushrooms and onion and cook until softened, about 5 minutes. Remove from heat and stir in remaining ingredients. Serve warm.

Makes about 1¼ cups.

QUESADILLA

2 corn tortillas
2 teaspoons margarine
¼ cup shredded cheddar cheese
1 tomato, halved
2 teaspoons finely chopped Bermuda
    onion

1. Preheat over to 400°F (205°C). Spread one side of each tortilla with one teaspoon margarine. Place on baking sheet.

2. On one-half of each tortilla arrange cheese, half tomato slice, and chopped onion.

3. Bake until cheese begins to melt. Fold tortillas in half and continue baking until edges are crisp. Serve hot.

Makes 1 to 2 servings.

FRUIT-NUT BUTTER

1½ cups cashews
½ cup raisins, chopped
½ cup sesame seeds

1. Grind cashews in blender. Add raisins and sesame seeds and blend well.

Makes about 2 cups.

AVOCADO SANDWICH

1 avocado, peeled and pitted
1 teaspoon finely chopped green
    onion
¼ teaspoon fresh lemon juice
¼ teaspoon chopped parsley leaves
⅛ teaspoon dill weed
⅛ teaspoon sea salt
Whole-grain bread
Alfalfa sprouts

1. Mash avocado in small bowl.

2. Blend in all remaining ingredients.

3. Spread on bread and top with sprouts.

Makes 1 to 2 servings.

CREAM CHEESE SANDWICH

2 slices whole-wheat raisin bread
Homemade cream cheese (page 109)
Walnuts, chopped
Dates, pitted and chopped
Apple slices
Banana slices

1. Spread bread generously with cream cheese.

2. Sprinkle one slice with walnuts, the other with dates.

3. Sandwich the two slices. Cut sandwich in half or fourths. Garnish with apple and banana slices.

Makes 1 to 2 servings.

MELTED NATURAL CHEDDAR SPECIAL SANDWICH

2 slices whole wheat or rye bread, halved
Cheddar cheese, grated
Sunflower seeds
Pumpkin seeds
Sesame seeds
Green onion, finely chopped
Lettuce
Cucumber
Tomato
Carrot
Parsley

1. Arrange bread on toasting pan or baking sheet.

2. Cover each piece with cheese. Sprinkle with sunflower, pumpkin, and sesame seeds. Top with small amount of green onion.

3. Toast until cheese melts. Serve hot. Garnish with fresh lettuce, cucumber, tomato, carrot, and parsley.

Makes 1 to 2 servings.

NUT BUTTER SANDWICH

Almond butter
Cashew butter
2 slices whole-wheat raisin bread
Dates, pitted and chopped
Banana slices
Sliced fresh fruit: apple, pear, etc.

1. Combine nut butters in desired proportions. Spread generously on bread.

2. Sprinkle one slice with dates. Top the other with banana slices.

3. Sandwich the two slices. Cut sandwich in half or fourths. Garnish with slices of fresh apple, pear, or other fruit.

Makes 1 to 2 servings.

BEVERAGES

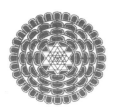

GRAPE-APPLE DRINK

1 cup apple juice
½ cup grape juice
¼ cup raisins
2 teaspoons brewer's yeast
1 teaspoon yogurt

Combine all ingredients in blender and blend until smooth.

Makes about 1¾ cups.

PINEAPPLE DRINK

1½ cups pineapple juice
1 banana, peeled and cut into several pieces
1 tablespoon yogurt
2 teaspoons wheat-germ powder
1 teaspoon sunflower seed meal

Combine all ingredients in blender and blend until smooth.

Makes about 2 cups.

FRUIT JUICE

1 cup coconut milk
¼ cup papaya juice
¼ cup pineapple juice
¼ cup orange juice

Combine all ingredients in 2-cup measure and stir to blend

Makes about 1¾ cups.

DATE-NUT SHAKE

1 cup milk
½ cup dates, pitted
1 tablespoon cashew or almond butter
1 tablespoon carob powder

Combine all ingredients in blender and blend until smooth.

Makes about 1½ cups.

FRUIT MILK

½ cup raw or nonfat milk
½ cup any fruit juice
½ teaspoon honey

Combine all ingredients in glass and stir to blend.

Makes about 1 cup.

ENERGY DRINK

½ cup prune juice
½ cup apple juice
1 teaspoon nut butter
1 teaspoon yogurt
1 teaspoon soy, sesame, or safflower oil

Combine all ingredients in blender and blend until smooth.

Makes about 1 cup.

OASIS SHAKE

1 cup milk
1 small banana, peeled and cut into several pieces
¼ cup coconut milk
3 pitted dates

Combine all ingredients in blender and blend until smooth.

Makes about 2 cups.

CAROB-HONEY SHAKE

½ small banana
1 cup milk
1 tablespoon carob powder
1 tablespoon sesame protein powder
1 tablespoon honey

Combine all ingredients in blender and blend until smooth.

Makes about 1½ cups.

CARROT MILK

½ cup carrot juice
½ cup milk
¼ cup chopped almonds
2 teaspoons wheat-germ powder

Combine all ingredients in blender and blend until smooth.

Makes about 1¼ cups.

CAROB MILK

2 cups milk
1 banana, peeled and cut into several
    pieces
2 tablespoons carob powder
1 tablespoon honey or molasses
1 tablespoon cashew or almond nut
    butter

Combine all ingredients in blender
and blend until smooth.

Makes about 2¾ cups.

POTASSIUM VEGETABLE DRINK

¼ cup parsley juice
¼ cup carrot juice
¼ cup celery juice
¼ cup watercress leaves
¼ cup coarsely chopped spinach
    leaves

Combine all ingredients in blender
and blend until smooth

Makes about 1¼ cups.

DATE MILK

1 cup milk
3 pitted dates
1 tablespoon shredded coconut
1 teaspoon wheat-germ powder
1 teaspoon safflower oil

Combine all ingredients in blender
and blend until smooth.

Makes about 1¼ cups.

GRAPE DRINK

1 cup grape juice
1 tablespoon brewer's yeast
1 tablespoon sunflower seed meal
1 tablespoon yogurt
1 teaspoon carob powder

Combine all ingredients in blender
and blend until smooth.

Makes about 1¼ cups.

VEGETABLE DRINK

½ cup tomato juice
¼ cup celery juice
¼ cup carrot juice
¼ cup watercress leaves
2 teaspoons brewer's yeast
1 teaspoon parsley leaves
1 teaspoon lemon juice

Combine all ingredients in blender
and blend until smooth.

Makes about 1¼ cups.

VEGETABLE-FRUIT JUICE

½ cup carrot juice
½ cup papaya juice or coconut milk
1 banana, peeled and cut into several
    pieces
2 pitted dates
1 tablespoon wheat germ

Combine all ingredients in blender
and blend until smooth.

Makes about 1½ cups.

VEGETABLE JUICE

⅓ cup beet juice
⅓ cup cucumber juice
⅓ cup carrot juice
1 tablespoon brewer's yeast

Combine all ingredients in blender
and blend until smooth.

Makes about 1 cup.

SALAD IN A GLASS

3 cups pure, unsalted tomato juice
2 tomatoes, coarsely chopped
½ cucumber, sliced
1 slice green pepper
½ stalk celery, sliced
1 green onion, sliced
3 sprigs fresh parsely

Combine all ingredients in blender
and blend until smooth.

Makes about 4 to 5 cups.

HOLIDAY PUNCH

1 quart apple juice
Juice of 6 oranges
3 cups cranberry juice
¼ cup lemon juice
½ cup honey
Orange slices studded with cloves,
        or cinnamon sticks (garnish)

To serve cold: Combine juices and
honey in punchbowl and stir to blend.
Garnish with orange slices.
To serve hot: Combine juices and
honey in 4-quart saucepan. Place
over medium heat until heated
through, stirring occasionally. Ladle
into mugs and garnish with cinnamon
sticks.

Makes 10 to 11 cups.

PINEAPPLE-COCONUT DRINK

½ cup coconut milk
½ cup pineapple juice
1 tablespoon yogurt
1 teaspoon wheat-germ powder

Combine all ingredients in blender
and blend until smooth.

Makes about 1 cup.

TOMATO DRINK

1 cup tomato juice
2 teaspoons brewer's yeast
1 teaspoon lemon juice
1 teaspoon parsley leaves

Combine all ingredients in blender
and blend until smooth.

Makes about 1 cup.

CARROT-COCONUT DRINK

½ cup carrot juice
¼ cup celery juice
¼ cup coconut milk
1 teaspoon parsley leaves
1 teaspoon brewer's yeast

Combine all ingredients in blender
and blend until smooth.

Makes about 1 cup.

VEGETABLE JUICE

⅓ cup carrot juice
⅓ cup celery juice
⅓ cup tomato juice
1 tablespoon brewer's yeast

Combine all ingredients in blender
and blend until smooth.

Makes about 1 cup.

FRUIT JUICE EGG DRINK

½ cup orange juice
½ cup papaya juice
1 egg
1 teaspoon honey

Combine all ingredients in blender
and blend until smooth.

Makes about 1¼ cups.

CAROB DRINK

1 cup milk
1 tablespoon carob powder
1 egg yolk
1 teaspoon wheat-germ powder
1 drop vanilla

Combine all ingredients in blender
and blend until smooth.

Makes about 1¼ cups.

APPLE DRINK

1 cup apple juice
1 tablespoon yogurt
1 to 2 teaspoons brewer's yeast
1 drop vanilla

Combine all ingredients in blender and blend until smooth.

Makes about 1 cup.

WEIGHT-GAINING DRINK

1 cup orange juice
1 egg
1 tablespoon Honey-Carrot Ice
    Cream (page 159)
1 tablespoon brewer's yeast
1 tablespoon cashew butter
1 teaspoon safflower oil

Combine all ingredients in blender and blend until smooth.

Makes about 2 cups.

PINEAPPLE-CARROT DRINK

½ cup pineapple juice
½ cup carrot juice
2 teaspoons brewer's yeast
1 teaspoon lemon juice
1 teaspoon shredded coconut

Combine all ingredients in blender and blend until smooth.

Makes about 1 cup.

HERB TEAS

1. Place 3 to 5 teaspoons of fresh or dried herbs in a preheated china or pottery teapot. For each teaspoonful of herb, bring 1 cup water to a rolling boil and pour into teapot.

2. Steep until tea is desired strength, about 5 minutes.

Some delicious teas are:

   Alfalfa leaves
   Camomile blossoms
   Sarsparilla
   Catnip
   Linden blossoms
   Rose hips
   Comfrey
   Hyssop
   Oat straw
   Mint
   Parsley
   Lavender blossoms
   Sassafras
   Fenugreek

Herbs can also be mixed in different combination.

COOL TEAS

1. Place 4 teaspoons herb or combination of herbs in 1-quart container. Fill container with spring or distilled water.

2. Let stand until tea is desired strength, several hours or overnight. Strain. Serve with honey, lemon, and sprig of mint.

LENTIL SOUP

¼ cup olive oil
1 onion, chopped
2 cloves garlic, minced
2 tomatoes, chopped
2 to 3 stalks celery with tops,
    chopped
2 or 3 carrots, chopped
1½ quarts water
2 cups lentils
1 tablespoon lemon juice
Savory
Thyme
Parsley
Oregano

1. Heat olive oil in large saucepan over medium heat. Add onion and cook until softened, about 5 minutes. Stir in garlic and cook 2 minutes.

2. Add chopped vegetables, water, lentils, lemon juice and herbs. Bring to boil, then reduce heat and simmer slowly until lentils are tender, about 2 hours.

3. Serve as is with whole lentils, or, for thicker soup, ladle a portion of soup into blender. Puree briefly and return to saucepan.

Makes 4 to 6 servings.

CROUTONS

¼ cup olive oil or margarine
1 clove garlic, minced
1 to 2 teaspoons minced herbs:
    marjoram, thyme, etc.
10 slices stale whole-grain bread, cut
    into ½-inch cubes

1. Preheat oven to 325°F (165°C). Heat oil in small skillet over medium heat. Add garlic and herbs and cook 3 minutes. Combine with bread cubes in large bowl and toss until evenly coated.

2. Spread on baking sheet and toast in oven until crisp and golden, about 15 to 20 minutes, stirring occasionally.

Use for garnishing soups or in salads.

YOGURT SOUP

1 pint yogurt
3 cucumbers, sliced
3 tablespoons soy oil
3 tablespoons lemon juice
1 tablespoon chopped mint
1 clove garlic, minced
1 teaspoon grated lemon rind
½ teaspoon dill weed
½ teaspoon dill seeds
Fresh dill sprigs (garnish)

1. Combine all ingredients in blender and puree until smooth.

2. Chill. Serve garnished with fresh dill.

Makes 3 to 4 servings.

MINESTRONE

1 cup beans: pea, marrow, or navy
6 cups water
¼ cup olive oil
1 onion, chopped
1 clove garlic, minced
2 tablespoons chopped celery
3 cups tomato juice or stock
1 cup chopped cabbage
½ cup vegetable or whole-wheat macaroni
2 tablespoons chopped parsley leaves
¼ teaspoon oregano
Vegetable salt, to taste
Parmesan cheese

1. Soak beans in water overnight. Simmer beans in soaking water until tender.

2. Heat oil in medium stockpot over medium heat. Add onion, garlic, and celery and cook until softened, about 5 minutes.

3. Add beans (with cooking liquid) and all remaining ingredients except cheese. Simmer 30 to 40 minutes.

4. Ladle into bowls, top with Parmesan and serve.

Makes 4 to 5 servings.

ONION SOUP

¼ cup oil
4 onions, chopped
1 stalk celery with leaves, chopped
2 cups stock (water in which vegetables were cooked or beans were soaked) or plain water
2 cups tomato juice
Vegetable salt, to taste
Garlic powder, to taste
1½- to 1-inch-thick slice whole-wheat bread
Margarine
Parmesan cheese

1. Heat oil in large saucepan over medium heat. Add onions and celery and cook until lightly browned, stirring frequently.

2. Add stock, juice, and seasonings. Bring to simmer, then cover and simmer over low heat, 15 minutes.

3. Spread bread with margarine; sprinkle with cheese. Cut slice in fourths. Place under broiler until browned.

4. Float one piece of cheese bread in each bowl of soup.

Makes 4 servings.

SPLIT PEA SOUP

1 quart water
1 cup split peas
1 large onion, chopped
4 carrots, chopped
2 stalks celery, chopped
¼ cup chopped parsley leaves
1 teaspoon soy oil or olive oil or margarine
1 teaspoon oregano
1 teaspoon basil
Vegetable salt, to taste

Combine all ingredients in 2-quart saucepan. Bring to boil, then reduce heat and simmer 2 hours.

If smoother consistency is desired, purée in blender.

Makes 3 to 4 servings.

EASY CREAM OF TOMATO SOUP

1 quart milk
2 cups stewed or pureed tomatoes
½ onion, chopped
3 tablespoons whole-wheat flour
1 teaspoon soy flour
Vegetable salt, to taste

1. Combine all ingredients in blender and puree until smooth.

2. Pour into large saucepan. Simmer soup 5 minutes, stirring. Serve hot.

Makes 4 to 5 servings.

VEGETABLE SOUP

¼ cup olive oil
1 large onion, chopped
3 fresh tomatoes, sliced
2 cloves garlic, minced
1 quart water
3 stalks celery with tops, chopped
3 carrots, sliced
2 cups chopped green beans
1 zucchini, cut in cubes
1 potato, cut in cubes
1 bay leaf
Marjoram, to taste
Parsley
Vegetable salt

1. Heat oil in large saucepan over medium heat. Add onion and cook until lightly browned.

2. Add tomatoes and garlic and simmer 5 minutes.

3. Add water and bring to boil.

4. Stir in vegetables and herbs. Bring to simmer; let simmer until vegetables are tender.

5. Season to taste with vegetable salt. Serve hot.

Makes 4 to 5 servings.

CHEESE AND BLACK BREAD SOUP

6 slices toasted pumpernickel or rye bread
½ pound grated Gruyere or Swiss cheese
1 quart milk
¼ cup butter
Dash of nutmeg

1. Place slice of toast in each bowl. Top with generous layer of cheese.

2. Bring milk to simmer. Remove from heat and skim. Add butter and nutmeg, stirring until butter melts. Pour around toast in each bowl. Serve immediately.

Makes 6 servings.

CREAM OF ZUCCHINI SOUP

4 zucchini or crookneck squash, cut into ½-inch slices
½ cup yogurt
1 tablespoon margarine
Vegetable salt

Combine zucchini in medium saucepan with enough water to cover. Simmer until tender. Transfer zucchini and cooking liquid to blender. Add yogurt and margarine and puree. Return to saucepan and thin with broth or water if necessary. Reheat, but do not boil. Season with vegetable salt.

Makes 3 to 4 servings.

GAZPACHO

3 cups tomato juice
3 tomatoes, peeled, seeded, and diced
1 cucumber, diced
1 green pepper, finely chopped
1 tablespoon chopped parsley leaves
1 clove garlic, mashed
1 tablespoon cider vinegar
Juice of 1 lemon
Vegetable salt, to taste
Avocado (garnish)

Combine all ingredients, except avocado, in large bowl, cover and chill thoroughly. Serve garnished with avocado.

Makes 4 to 5 servings.

JACK O'LANTERN PUMPKIN SOUP

1 10- to 12-inch-diameter pumpkin
3 cups toasted whole-wheat bread crumbs
¾ pound Gruyere or Swiss cheese, sliced
Vegetable salt, to taste
Freshly ground nutmeg
Milk

1. Preheat oven to 350° (175°C). Cut lid in pumpkin, jack o'lantern style. Remove seeds and fibrous membranes. Alternate layers of bread crumbs and cheese inside pumpkin, seasoning with vegetable salt and nutmeg.

2. Pour in milk to within 1 inch of top of pumpkin. Replace lid. Set pumpkin in roasting pan and bake until tender, about 1 hour. Check midway during baking and add more milk if necessary.

3. Serve hot from pumpkin, scooping bits of pumpkin meat with soup.

Makes 6 servings.

BLACK BEAN SOUP

½ pound black beans
6 cups water
2 tablespoons olive oil
1 small onion, chopped
½ green pepper, chopped
1 stalk celery, chopped
1 clove garlic, minced
½ teaspoon thyme
½ teaspoon oregano

1. Soak beans overnight.

2. Heat oil in medium stockpot over medium heat. Add onion, green pepper, and celery and cook until tender, 7 to 10 minutes. Add garlic and herbs, reduce heat to low and cook 3 minutes.

3. Blend in beans (with soaking liquid). Simmer until beans are so tender they begin to fall apart. Strain soup or puree in blender. Serve hot.

Makes 4 to 6 servings.

STRACCIATELLA

6 cups stock
2 bunches spinach leaves, shredded
2 eggs, beaten
¼ cup whole-wheat bread crumbs
¼ cup grated Parmesan cheese

1. Bring stock to simmer in large saucepan. Add spinach and simmer 3 minutes.

2. Combine eggs, crumbs, and cheese. Bring stock to boil and stir in egg mixture. Serve immediately.

Makes 4 to 6 servings.

CABBAGE AND POTATO SOUP

1 quart water
1 onion, chopped
Vegetable salt, to taste
3 potatoes, peeled and sliced
½ pound cabbage, finely shredded
½ cup olive oil or margarine

1. Combine water, onion, and vegetable salt in medium stockpot and bring to boil.

2. Add potatoes and simmer until tender.

3. Remove potatoes using slotted spoon. Force through ricer, then return to soup. Add cabbage and oil and simmer 3 to 4 minutes. Serve hot.

Makes 4 to 5 servings.

CREAM OF BROCCOLI SOUP

2 pounds broccoli, coarsely chopped
1 onion, chopped
1 bay leaf
1 cup milk
Vegetable salt, to taste
Nutmeg, to taste
Chopped chives or sesame seeds

1. Combine broccoli, onion, and bay leaf in medium stockpot. Cover with water, bring to simmer, and cook until tender.

2. Strain liquid, adding water if necessary to make 2 cups.

3. Transfer liquid and vegetables to blender and puree until smooth.

4. Return to stockpot and stir in milk. Add seasonings and heat through.

5. Ladle into bowls and sprinkle with chopped chives or sesame seeds. Serve hot.

Makes 4 to 5 servings.

CREAM OF SPINACH SOUP

2 tablespoons margarine
1 onion, chopped
1 quart milk
Vegetable salt, to taste
2 cups finely chopped or liquefied
spinach leaves
Chopped parsley leaves

1. Melt margarine in large saucepan over medium heat. Add onion and cook until transparent, 7 to 10 minutes.

2. Add 3 cups milk and vegetable salt. Bring to simmer, then add spinach and simmer 3 more minutes.

3. Transfer to blender and puree until smooth. Return to saucepan and add remaining 1 cup milk. Heat through.

4. Ladle into bowls and sprinkle with parsley. Serve hot.

Makes 4 to 5 servings.

FRESH TOMATO PURÉE

6 to 8 ripe plum tomatoes, peeled, seeded, and chopped
1 tablespoon margarine

Combine tomatoes and margarine in saucepan. Bring to simmer; let simmer until smooth and thickened, stirring frequently.

If smoother sauce is desired, puree in blender.

Makes 1 to 1½ cups.

FRESH PEA SOUP

3 cups shelled peas
2 cups water
¼ cup chopped green onions
3 tablespoons margarine
3 tablespoons whole wheat flour
3 cups milk
Chives or mint leaves, chopped

1. Simmer peas in water until tender. Transfer peas and cooking liquid to blender. Add onion and puree.

2. Melt margarine in 2-quart saucepan over low heat. Add flour and cook, stirring, 3 minutes. Slowly stir in milk and cook until mixture thickens. Blend in pureed peas.

3. Chill. Serve with sprinkled chives or mint.

Makes 3 to 4 servings.

POTATO SOUP

¼ cup margarine
1 onion, chopped
1 teaspoon paprika
1 quart water
4 pounds potatoes, peeled and sliced
2 cups milk
Celery salt

1. Melt margarine in large saucepan over medium heat. Add onion and paprika and cook until onion is transparent, 7 to 10 minutes. Add water and bring to boil.

2. Add potatoes. Reduce heat and simmer uncovered until potatoes are tender.

3. Stir in milk and cook until potatoes fall apart. Transfer soup to blender and puree until smooth. Season to taste with celery salt. Serve hot.

4. For an interesting variation stir ½ pound grated Monterey Jack cheese into hot soup just before serving.

Makes 8 to 10 servings.

BARLEY SOUP

¼ cup margarine
2 onions, chopped
4 carrots, chopped
1 turnip, chopped
7 cups water
1 cup pearl barley
Milk, warmed (optional)
Vegetable salt, to taste
Chopped parsley leaves

1. Melt margarine in medium stock-pot over medium heat. Add onions, carrots, and turnip and cook until softened, 7 to 10 minutes.

2. Add water and bring to boil. Stir in barley. Cover and simmer gently 2 hours.

3. Thin soup with warm milk if necessary. Season with vegetable salt. Ladle into bowls and sprinkle with parsley. Serve hot.

Makes 4 to 6 servings

CORN CHOWDER

2 cups cubed potatoes
2 tablespoons margarine or oil
½ onion, chopped
Kernels from 3 ears of corn
¼ teaspoon paprika
¼ teaspoon savory
¼ teaspoon celery salt
Vegetable salt, to taste

1. Combine potatoes with enough water to cover in medium saucepan and simmer until tender.

2. Melt margarine in large skillet over medium heat. Add onion and cook until golden. Add potatoes (with water) and all remaining ingredients.

3. Simmer 15 to 20 minutes, stirring occasionally. Serve hot.

Makes 4 servings.

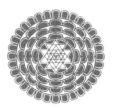

SPROUTS

1. Place correct quantity of seeds in 1-quart jar. Stretch cheesecloth over top and secure with rubber band. Cover seeds with warm water. Let stand overnight.

2. In the morning, pour off water and rinse with clean water.

3. Place jar on its side in a dark cupboard.

4. Rinse sprouts 3 to 4 times daily, swirling water around in jar and pouring off through cheesecloth.

5. When sprouts have grown to suggested length, remove cheesecloth, cover with lid and refrigerate.

Seed	Amount (For 1-quart jar)	Number of Days	Suggested Length
Alfalfa	3 tablespoons	4	2 inches
Lentil	½ cup	3	½ to 1 inch
Wheat	1 cup	2	¼ to ½ inch
Sunflower	1 cup	2	¼ inch
Mung beans	½ cup	3	2 inches
Radish	¼ cup	3	1 inch

ROMAINE SALAD

1 head romaine lettuce, torn
¼ cup olive oil
¼ cup Parmesan cheese
Vegetable salt
¼ cup lemon juice
1 cup whole-wheat croutons

Place romaine in salad bowl. Add all remaining ingredients in order listed and toss thoroughly. Serve immediately.

Makes 4 to 6 servings.

LENTIL SPROUT SALAD

2 bunches fresh spinach leaves, torn
1 large red apple (unpeeled), cored, quartered, and thinly sliced
1 cup lentil sprouts
½ Bermuda onion, thinly sliced
3 tablespoons olive oil
2 tablespoons lemon juice
1 teaspoon Fines Herbes
Vegetable salt, to taste

1. Combine spinach, apple, sprouts, and onion in salad bowl.

2. Combine oil, lemon juice, herbs, and vegetable salt in small bowl and whisk to blend.

3. Pour over salad and toss well.

Makes 4 to 6 servings.

BROCCOLI SALAD

3 cups fresh broccoli florets, lightly
    steamed
1 cup cherry tomatoes, halved
½ Bermuda onion, thinly sliced
1 teaspoon chopped fresh basil
Kelp Dressing (p. 131)

Combine broccoli, tomatoes, onion,
and basil in salad bowl. Add Kelp
Dressing as desired and toss to blend.
Serve immediately.

Makes 4 to 6 servings.

GREEN BEAN SALAD

2 cups crisp, raw green beans
3 bunches spinach leaves, torn
¼ head Boston lettuce, torn
2 tomatoes, sliced
½ Bermuda onion, thinly sliced
Kelp (p. 131) or Blender Herb
    Dressing (p. 130)

Remove strings from beans. Snap
each bean into 3 or 4 pieces. Combine beans, greens, tomatoes, and
onion in salad bowl. Add dressing
as desired and toss to blend. Serve
immediately.

Makes 4 to 6 servings.

RAW PEA SALAD

1 cup fresh raw peas
2 cups grated carrots
1 cup sunflower seeds
1 green onion, chopped
Dressing as desired

Combine all ingredients in salad
bowl. Add dressing and toss well.

Makes 4 to 6 servings.

KIDNEY, GARBANZO, AND GREEN BEAN SALAD

1½ cups cooked kidney beans
1½ cups cooked garbanzo beans
2 cups freshly steamed green beans
½ clove garlic, minced
½ Bermuda or Spanish onion,
    chopped
½ cup olive oil
½ cup cider vinegar
1 teaspoon basil
1 teaspoon oregano
Lettuce leaves
Tomato wedges

Combine beans, garlic, and onion in
salad bowl. Add oil, vinegar, and
herbs, and toss well. Serve on lettuce
leaves with tomato wedges.

Makes 6 servings.

SPINACH SALAD

1 pound raw spinach, torn
1 onion, grated
1 clove garlic, minced
7 tablespoons oil
2 tablespoons lemon juice
Tomato wedges
¼ cup tofu, chopped

Place spinach in salad bowl. Blend
onion, garlic, oil, and lemon juice.
Pour over spinach and toss well. Top
with tomato and tofu.

Makes 4 to 6 servings.

TOSSED GREEN SALAD

1 head lettuce
1 large bunch watercress leaves
1 head curly escarole
2 Belgian endives, sliced
2 cucumbers, sliced
Natural Herb Dressing (p. 130)
3 tomatoes, cut in wedges
2 tablespoons grated lemon peel

Combine greens and cucumbers in
salad bowl. Add dressing and toss
well. Top with tomatoes and sprinkle
with lemon peel.

Makes 4 to 6 servings.

GREEK SALAD

1 head romaine or iceberg lettuce,
   torn
2 tomatoes, cut into wedges
5 green onions, chopped
15 Greek olives, pitted and halved
10 radishes, sliced
¼ pound feta cheese (optional)
¼ cup lemon juice
¼ cup olive oil
¼ teaspoon oregano
Vegetable salt

1. Place lettuce in salad bowl.

2. Add tomatoes, green onions, olives,
and radishes.

3. Crumble feta cheese over salad.

4. Combine lemon juice, oil, oregano
and vegetable salt in small bowl and
whisk to blend.

5. Pour over salad and toss well.

Makes 4 to 6 servings

EGYPTIAN SALAD

1 cup yogurt
1 teaspoon fresh dill, finely chopped
½ teaspoon garlic, finely chopped
4 cucumbers, peeled, halved lengthwise, and thinly sliced
3 radishes, thinly sliced

Blend yogurt, dill, and garlic in salad
bowl. Add cucumber and radish
slices, and toss well. Chill before
serving.

Makes 4 to 6 servings.

CUCUMBER SALAD

2 to 3 cucumbers, thinly sliced
1 cup yogurt
3 tablespoons chopped green onions
3 tablespoons lemon juice
½ teaspoon dill weed

Combine all ingredients in salad
bowl. Chill before serving.

Makes 4 to 6 servings.

BEET SALAD

Young, tender beets (uncooked)
Lemon juice
Honey
Oil

Trim and peel beets. Grate beets or
finely chop. Chill thoroughly. To
serve, dress with lemon juice, honey,
and oil to taste.

TOFU (Bean Cake)

3 cups soybeans
3 teaspoons nigari or epsom salts
   (Nigari is available in Oriental
   markets. If unavailable, epsom
   salts can be substituted.)

1. Soak soybeans in water to cover
overnight.

2. Drain. Transfer 1 cup soybeans to
blender with 2 cups fresh water; liq-
uefy. Repeat until all soybeans are
liquefied.

3. Set colander over clean large pot
and line colander with clean 2-foot-
square piece of cotton fabric (a piece
of old sheet will serve the purpose).
Pour in soybean mixture. Gather up
the edges and squeeze soy milk
through cloth into pot. Add pulp to
soy milk in pot and add 1 quart
water. Mix and squeeze again.

4. Measure soy milk into 8- to 10-
quart pot. Add boiling water to make
6 quarts. Bring to boil, stirring. Simmer 7 minutes.

5. Remove from heat.

6. Dissolve nigari in 1½ cups water.
Slowly stir into soy milk, one-third
at a time. Cover and let stand 2 to
3 minutes.

7. Line colander with damp cotton cloth. Ladle in curds. Fold edges of cloth over curds and top with plate or bowl. Let stand 30 minutes, then remove plate. Tofu is ready for use.

Unused tofu should be covered with water and refrigerated. If water is changed daily, tofu will remain fresh for 1 week.

BEAN SPROUT SALAD

¼ pound mung bean sprouts
Celery, chopped
Pecans or walnuts, chopped
Caraway seeds
Honey
Lemon juice
Lettuce leaves

Combine bean sprouts, celery, and nuts. Mix in enough caraway seeds to add delicate flavor. Add honey and lemon juice to taste, and toss to blend. Serve on lettuce leaves.

Makes 4 to 6 servings.

EGGPLANT SALAD

½ eggplant, trimmed
½ cauliflower, trimmed and thinly sliced
4 bunches spinach, torn
2 yellow summer squash, thinly sliced
½ Bermuda onion, thinly sliced
½ cup bean sprouts
¼ cup pumpkin seeds
Blender or Natural Herb Dressing (p. 130)

1. Cut eggplant into 3 to 4 lengthwise slices, then crosswise into ⅛-inch-thick slices.

2. Combine with remaining vegetables, sprouts, and seeds in salad bowl. Add herb dressing and toss well.

Makes 6 to 8 servings.

LEEK SALAD

1 clove garlic, split
1 head romaine lettuce, torn
3 young, tender leeks, trimmed and sliced
1 tomato, sliced
Chervil
Basil
3 tablespoons olive oil
2 tablespoons lemon juice

Rub salad bowl with garlic. Add romaine, leeks, tomato, and herbs. Add oil and lemon juice and toss well.

Makes 4 to 6 servings

GUACAMOLE

1 avocado, peeled and pitted
1 tablespoon finely chopped onion, or to taste
1 clove garlic, minced
1 to 2 teaspoons lemon juice
1 to 2 teaspoons olive oil
Lettuce
Wheat crackers

Mash avocado in bowl. Blend in onion, garlic, lemon juice and olive oil. Serve on lettuce with crisp wheat crackers.

Makes 1 to 2 servings.

COMBINATION SALAD

1 medium-size head lettuce, shredded
1 bunch spinach, shredded
2 tomatoes, chopped
1 cucumber, finely chopped
1 green pepper, finely chopped
3 stalks celery, finely chopped
A few watercress leaves, chopped
Lemon juice
Oil
Honey

Combine vegetables in salad bowl. Add lemon juice, honey, and oil to taste and toss well.

Makes 4 to 6 servings.

DANDELION SALAD

1 clove garlic, split
1 pound tender dandelion greens
¾ cup black olives
1 ripe tomato, cut in eighths
Olive oil
Lemon juice

Rub salad bowl with garlic. Add greens, olives, and tomato. Add oil and lemon juice to taste and toss well.

Makes 4 to 6 servings.

COTTAGE CHEESE SALAD

1 cup mung bean sprouts
4 radishes, thinly sliced
¼ small cucumber, thinly sliced
2 green onions, thinly sliced
½ cup cottage cheese
½ cup yogurt

Combine sprouts and vegetables in salad bowl. Add cheese and yogurt and blend well. Chill before serving.

Makes 4 to 6 servings

HERB GARDEN COTTAGE CHEESE

1 pound cottage cheese
¼ cup yogurt
¼ cup poppy seeds
¼ cup caraway seeds
¼ cup sesame seeds
1 teaspoon minced chives
1 sprig of each, minced: marjoram, basil, thyme, sage, parsley, dill
Garlic powder

Blend all ingredients. Refrigerate 1 hour or more before serving.

Makes 4 to 6 servings.

HOMEMADE COTTAGE CHEESE

4 quarts (1 gallon) milk will make 1½ to 2 pounds of cheese. Place raw milk (cow or goat) in covered bowl and let stand in warm place until clabbered (24 to 36 hours). To firm curd, heat to 110°F (43°C). Strain through cheesecloth. Let drain.

AVOCADO ON THE HALF SHELL

Avocados, halved and pitted
Olive oil
Lemon juice

Spoon olive oil and lemon juice to taste into avocado cavities.

Serve one half per person.

COLESLAW

1 small head cabbage, shredded
6 tablespoons yogurt
2 tablespoons mayonnaise, preferably homemade
2 tablespoons lemon juice
1 tablespoon milk
Vegetable salt
Celery salt
Dill weed

Mix all ingredients well. Chill before serving.

Makes 4 to 6 servings.

POTATO SALAD

2 pounds potatoes
1 onion, thinly sliced
5 tablespoons olive oil
¼ cup cider vinegar
Vegetable salt, to taste
1 cup mayonnaise
3 hard-boiled eggs, sliced
¼ cup chopped ripe olives

1. Boil potatoes in water to cover until tender.

2. Peel and cut into thin slices or cubes.

3. Combine warm potatoes with onion, oil, vinegar, and vegetable salt. Add mayonnaise, eggs, and olives and blend well. Chill before serving.

Makes 4 to 6 servings.

INDIA NUT SALAD

1 head Boston lettuce, torn
2 cups chopped pecans or walnuts
8 dates, pitted and chopped
¼ cup shredded coconut
1 red apple (unpeeled), cored and
    sliced
3 tablespoons raisins
French Dressing (p. 131)

Combine all ingredients in salad
bowl and toss well.

Makes 4 to 6 servings

PAPAYA-PINEAPPLE SALAD

2 papayas, peeled, seeded, and
    coarsely chopped (reserve seeds
    for dressing)
1 banana, sliced
½ pineapple, coarsely chopped
¼ cup honey
3 tablespoons lemon juice
Papaya Seed Dressing (p. 130)

Mix all fruits. Blend in honey and
lemon juice. Serve with Papaya Seed
Dressing.

Makes 4 to 6 servings.

CHEESE AND CELERY SALAD

1 cup (8 ounces) cream cheese
1 to 2 tablespoons milk
1 cup chopped celery
1 tablespoon chopped green onion
Celery salt
Watercress, lettuce, or celery stalks

Blend cheese and milk. Add celery
and green onion. Season with dash
of celery salt. Serve on watercress
or lettuce, or use as a filling for celery stalks.

Makes 4 to 6 servings.

RAW VEGETABLE STICKS

Wash and slice into finger-sized sticks
any or all of the following:

Broccoli
Carrots
Celery
Green onion
Zucchini
Cauliflower
Cucumbers
Eggplant
Turnip
Bermuda onion
Bell pepper
Radishes
Rutabaga
Whole cherry tomatoes

Dip in yogurt or guacamole.

PEAR SALAD

4 pears
French Dressing (p.131)
1 cup cottage cheese

1. Combine pears (whole or halves)
and French Dressing and marinate
in refrigerator several hours.

2. Mound cottage cheese on platter.
Arrange pears around cheese. Pour
additional dressing over all and serve.

Makes 4 servings.

CANTALOUPE CUP

1 small cantaloupe, halved and
    seeded
1 to 2 cups berries or chopped sea-
    sonal fruit
Yogurt, honey, or shredded coconut

Fill cantaloupe halves with fruit. Top
with yogurt, honey, or coconut.

Makes 2 servings.

WATERCRESS AND GRAPEFRUIT SALAD

3 sweet grapefruits, peeled, seeded, and sectioned
1 to 2 bunches watercress, torn
French Dressing (p. 131)
Honey

Combine grapefruit sections and watercress in bowl. Add French Dressing as desired, and toss well. Sweeten lightly with honey.

Makes 4 to 6 servings.

ENDIVE AND ORANGE SALAD

2 to 3 Belgian endives, halved
2 to 3 oranges, peeled and thinly sliced
Lettuce or watercress
French Dressing (p. 131)

Arrange endive and orange slices atop lettuce or watercress on individual plates. Pour on French Dressing as desired.

Makes 4 to 6 servings.

FRESH FRUIT SALAD

1 cup sliced bananas, tossed with lemon juice to prevent darkening
1 cup strawberries
1 cup sliced peaches
½ cup freshly grated coconut
¼ cup chopped almonds or pignolias
Honey to taste

Combine all ingredients.

Makes 4 to 6 servings.

APPLE SALAD

4 apples, grated
½ pound almonds, ground
¾ cup raisins
Nutmeg, to taste

Combine all ingredients.

Makes 6 servings.

DRIED FRUIT SALAD

1 cup chopped, pitted dates
1 cup chopped figs
1 cup raisins
1 cup grated coconut
Yogurt
Honey

Combine fruits and coconut. Add yogurt and honey as desired and toss well.

Makes 4 to 6 servings.

WALDORF SALAD

2 tart, crisp apples, diced
1 cup chopped celery
½ cup pecans
½ cup raisins
Mayonnaise, preferably homemade
Lettuce

Combine apples, celery, pecans, and raisins with enough mayonnaise to moisten. Serve on lettuce leaves.

Makes 4 to 6 servings.

CARROT SALAD

3 cups grated carrots
½ cup raisins
¾ cup fresh or frozen pineapple chunks
⅓ cup mayonnaise, preferably homemade

Combine all ingredients and toss well.

Makes 4 to 6 servings.

WINTER SALAD

3 apples, cored
1 banana
2 stalks celery
¼ cup raisins
10 pecans or walnuts
Mayonnaise, preferably homemade
Yogurt

Chop all ingredients and combine in bowl. Moisten with equal amounts of mayonnaise and yogurt and toss well.

Makes 4 to 6 servings.

TANGERINE-WATERCRESS SALAD

5 to 6 tangerines or 3 to 4 oranges, peeled, seeded and diced
2 bunches watercress leaves
¼ cup olive oil
2 teaspoons cider vinegar
1 teaspoon lemon juice
1 teaspoon honey

Combine all ingredients and toss well.

Makes 4 to 6 servings.

DRESSINGS

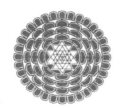

TOMATO-BASIL DRESSING

1 tomato, sliced
¼ cup olive oil, or mixture of safflower and olive oils
2 tablespoons lemon juice
6 to 8 fresh basil leaves
Vegetable salt
Garlic powder

Combine all ingredients in blender and blend until smooth.

Makes about ¾ cup.

MAYONNAISE

2 cups safflower, soy, olive, or sunflower oil
2 egg yolks
¼ cup lemon juice
1 to 2 teaspoons honey
1 teaspoon vegetable salt
¼ teaspoon dry mustard

Measure oil into pitcher or another container that is easy to pour from.

1. Combine all remaining ingredients in blender or small mixer bowl, and blend.

2. Continue blending or beating while adding oil drop by drop. If oil is added too fast, mayonnaise will not thicken. Stop adding oil when mayonnaise reaches desired consistency, even if all oil is not used.

3. Store in refrigerator.

Makes about 2 cups.

BLENDER HERB DRESSING

¼ cup chopped watercress or
   spinach
¼ cup oil
2 tablespoons lemon juice or cider
   vinegar
2 tablespoons chopped green onion
1 teaspoon honey
1 teaspoon savory
1 teaspoon parsley
1 teaspoon tarragon
1 teaspoon dill weed

Combine all ingredients in blender
and blend until smooth.

Makes about ¾ cup.

PAPAYA SEED DRESSING

2 cups safflower oil
½ cup honey
½ cup lemon juice
2 tablespoons fresh papaya seeds
Mint leaves

Combine all ingredients in blender
and blend until smooth.

Serve on fruit salads.

Makes about 3 cups.

YOGURT FRUIT SALAD DRESSING

1 cup yogurt
2 tablespoons lemon juice
2 tablespoons honey

Combine all ingredients and beat
well. Chill before serving.

Makes about 1¼ cups.

SESAME SEED DRESSING

½ cup olive oil
1 clove garlic, minced
2 teaspoons sesame seeds
3 tablespoons lemon juice
Vegetable salt, to taste

1. Heat oil in small skillet over medium heat. Add garlic and sesame
seeds and cook lightly.

2. Cool. Transfer to covered jar. Add
lemon juice and vegetable salt and
shake well.

Makes about ¾ cup.

TAHINI DRESSING

½ cup tahini (sesame butter)
¼ cup oil
Juice of ½ lemon
1 teaspoon thyme
1 teaspoon tamari (soy sauce)
½ teaspoon powdered kelp

Combine all ingredients in blender
and blend until smooth.

Makes about ¾ cup.

NATURAL HERB DRESSING

1⅓ cups olive oil
⅔ cup lemon juice
1 clove garlic (optional), minced
¼ teaspoon anise seeds
¼ teaspoon dill weed
¼ teaspoon mint
¼ teaspoon tarragon
¼ teaspoon *fine herbes* (sold at most
   stores carrying a good selection of
   herbs and spices; or make your
   own using an equal combination
   of sage, oregano, thyme, basil,
   marjoram and rosemary)

Combine oil, lemon juice, and garlic in covered jar. Finely crush anise
seeds and herbs. Add to oil mixture.
Shake well and use on any green
salad. Store in refrigerator.

Makes about 2 cups.

YOGURT DRESSING

1 cup plain yogurt
2 tablespons lemon juice
1 clove garlic, minced
¼ onion, grated
½ teaspoon paprika

Combine all ingredients and beat well. Chill before serving.

Makes about 1 cup.

AVOCADO DRESSING

1 avocado, peeled, pitted, and
   mashed
1 clove garlic, mashed
1 green onion, finely chopped
Milk

Combine avocado, garlic, and green onion. Thin slightly with milk. Serve immediately.

Makes about ½ cup.

COTTAGE CHEESE DRESSING

Place amount of cottage cheese needed in blender and blend at high speed for 5 minutes.

FRENCH DRESSING

¾ cup vegetable oil
¼ cup lemon juice
1 to 3 teaspoons honey
1 clove garlic, minced
1 teaspoon vegetable salt

Combine all ingredients in covered jar and shake well.

Makes about 1 cup.

KELP DRESSING

2 cups olive oil
Juice of 1 lemon
½ teaspoon powdered kelp
Vegetable salt, to taste

Combine all ingredients in covered jar and shake well.

Makes about 2 cups.

THOUSAND ISLAND DRESSING

1 cup olive oil
1 cup tomato puree
⅓ cup lemon juice
¼ cup honey
¼ onion, finely chopped

Combine all ingredients in covered jar and shake well.

Makes about 2½ cups.

TOMATO DRESSING

½ cup soy oil
¼ cup lemon juice
¼ cup tomato juice (if possible,
   make your own in your vegetable
   juice extractor)
Vegetable salt, to taste

Combine all ingredients in covered jar and shake well.

Makes about 1 cup.

MAIN DISHES

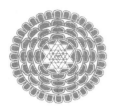

VEGETABLE CURRY

1 potato
2 bell peppers
1 large eggplant
2 zucchini
¼ cup margarine or oil
1 teaspoon ground ginger
1 teaspoon sea salt
½ teaspoon ground coriander
1 teaspoon mustard seeds
1 teaspoon cumin seeds
1 clove garlic, minced
3 or 4 tomatoes, cut into wedges

1. Cut potato, peppers, eggplant, and zucchini into bite-sized chunks.

2. Melt margarine in large skillet over medium heat. Add spices and garlic and sauté 3 minutes.

3. Add vegetables (except tomatoes) and cook, stirring frequently, 10 to 15 minutes. Add water if necessary to keep mixture moist.

4. When vegetables are tender, add tomatoes and heat through. Serve immediately.

STEAMED BEAN SPROUTS

1 tablespoon oil or margarine
1 onion, chopped
¼ cup water
4 cups bean sprouts
Soy sauce (optional)

1. Heat oil in large skillet over medium heat. Add onion and sauté until softened.

2. Add water, then sprouts. Steam very briefly, just until sprouts begin to wilt.

3. Add small dash of soy sauce, if desired. Serve immediately.

TOFU AND ONIONS

¼ cup oil
3 onions, sliced
1 pound tofu, drained and cut into 1-inch cubes
1½ teaspoons cornstarch
1½ teaspoons tamari (soy sauce)
¾ cup water

1. Heat oil in large skillet over medium heat. Add onions and sauté until wilted.

2. Stir in tofu.

3. Mix cornstarch and soy sauce until smooth. Blend in water. Add to skillet.

4. Simmer, stirring, until sauce is thickened. Serve hot.

CHINESE VEGETABLES

¼ cup oil
1 cup thinly sliced onions.
1 cup chopped green peppers
1 cup chopped celery and tops
½ cup sliced mushrooms
1 cup mung bean sprouts

1. Heat oil in large skillet over medium heat. Add onions, green peppers, celery, and mushrooms and sauté briefly.

2. Remove from heat, stir in sprouts, and serve.

LEMON RICE

3 tablespoons margarine
1 teaspoon black mustard seeds
3 cups cooked brown rice
¼ teaspoon saffron
Juice of 1 lemon

1. Melt margarine in medium saucepan over medium heat. Add mustard seeds and cook until they start to pop.

2. Add rice and saffron.

3. Cook, stirring, until heated through. Add lemon juice and serve.

PEA PODS AND BEAN SPROUTS

3 tablespoons oil
1 large onion, chopped
½ green pepper, chopped
1 stalk celery, chopped
2 pounds snow peas, trimmed
1 pound fresh bean sprouts
1 cup water
1 tablespoon soy sauce
1½ teaspoons arrowroot
1 cup tofu (optional), diced

1. Heat oil in large skillet over medium heat. Add onion, pepper, and celery and sauté until tender.

2. Add pea pods, bean sprouts and ½ cup water. Cover and steam 7 to 8 minutes.

3. Combine soy sauce, arrowroot, and remaining ½ cup water. Pour over vegetables and cook a few minutes longer to thicken sauce, stirring occasionally.

4. Tofu can be added if desired.

EGGPLANT ROLLS

1 cup grated Monterey Jack cheese
½ cup grated Parmesan cheese
⅓ cup ricotta cheese
1 egg, separated
1 tablespoon chopped parsley leaves
½ teaspoon oregano
Vegetable salt
⅓ cup milk
1 whole egg
2 tablespoons whole-wheat flour
5 tablespoons olive oil
½ teaspoon baking powder
1 large eggplant
Additional whole-wheat flour

1. Combine cheeses, 1 egg yolk (save the white), parsley, oregano, and a pinch of vegetable salt. Blend well.

2. Combine milk, whole egg, flour, 1 tablespoon of oil, and baking powder. Blend well to form batter.

3. Preheat oven to 375°F (190°C). Peel the eggplant; halve lengthwise. Cut lengthwise slices, about 1/16 inch thick. Flour slices lightly and dip into batter. Brown in remaining olive oil, and drain on paper towels.

4. Spoon dollop of cheese mixture onto each slice, and roll up.

5. Arrange rolls in oiled baking dish. Bake until cheese melts. Serve hot.

VEGETABLE TOFU KEBABS

1 cup butter or margarine
½ cup water
½ cup lemon juice
¼ cup tamari (soy sauce)
1 teaspoon curry powder
1 clove garlic, minced
Hard tofu
Any or all of the following vegetables, cut to appropriate size: zucchini, mushrooms, new potatoes, onions, eggplant, tomatoes, bell peppers
Cooked brown rice

1. Combine butter, water, lemon juice, soy sauce, curry powder, and garlic in medium saucepan and place over low heat until butter is melted.

2. Preheat oven to 350°F (175°C). Thread tofu and desired vegetables on skewers. Arrange in baking pan. Pour butter mixture over. Bake until vegetables are tender, about 1 hour, turning occasionally. Serve on brown rice, spooning sauce over.

STEAMED BROCCOLI

Rinse broccoli. Tie in bunches and stand up in deep kettle. Add water to come ¼ up stalks. Cover tightly and steam until tender.

GREEN BEANS IN HERB SAUCE

2 tablespoons oil
1 onion, sliced
1 tomato, cut in pieces
1 clove garlic, minced
1 tablespoon chopped celery
1 tablespoon minced green pepper
1 tablespoon chopped parsley leaves
¼ teaspoon savory
1 whole clove
2 pounds green beans, lightly
    steamed

1. Heat oil in medium skillet over medium heat. Add onion and sauté until tender.

2. Add all remaining ingredients except beans. Cover and simmer gently 10 minutes.

3. Pour mixture over beans. Serve hot.

BAKED CAULIFLOWER

1 large cauliflower
Whole-wheat bread crumbs
Margarine
Seasoning, to taste
1 cup milk

1. Steam cauliflower until crisp-tender. Slice.

2. Preheat oven to 350°F (175°C). Alternate layers of cauliflower and whole-wheat bread crumbs (toasted, if desired) in oiled casserole. Dot each layer with margarine and season as desired. Continue until cauliflower is used, with top layer bread crumbs. Pour milk over.

3. Bake until brown. Serve hot.

CELERIAC CASSEROLE

1 pound celeriac (celery root), thinly
    sliced
¼ pound shredded cheese
1 cup hot milk
3 tablespoons margarine
Vegetable salt, to taste

1. Preheat oven to 350°F (175°C). Alternate layers of celeriac and cheese in oiled baking dish. Pour hot milk over. Dot with margarine.

2. Bake until celeriac is tender, about 30 to 40 minutes. Serve hot. Season with salt to taste.

EGG FOO YUNG

2½ cups water
¼ cup soy sauce
1½ tablespoons arrowroot
6 to 8 eggs, beaten
¼ cup minced water chestnuts
3 stalks celery with tops, minced
3 green onions, minced
1 tablespoon honey
1 cup bean sprouts
¼ cup margarine

1. To make Chinese gravy blend water, soy sauce, and arrowroot. Cook over low heat until clear.

2. Combine eggs, minced vegetables and honey. (This can be done quickly in blender: Break eggs into blender container, adding vegetables cut in pieces, and honey. Blend, using "medium" or "chop" blender speed, for 10 seconds.)

3. Add bean sprouts to egg mixture. Melt margarine in large skillet. Pour in ¼ cup egg mixture for each patty.

4. Sauté over medium heat until browned. Turn and brown second side. Serve plain or with Chinese gravy.

RICE STUFFED PEPPERS

5 tablespoons olive oil
1 minced raw onion
2 tablespoons chopped parsley
1 clove garlic, minced
1 cup steamed brown rice
Sage
Thyme
6 large bell peppers
2 cups tomato puree

1. Heat ¼ cup oil in medium skillet over medium heat. Add onion, parsley, and garlic and sauté until tender.

2. Preheat oven to 350°F (175°C). Mix rice, herbs, and sautéed vegetables. Cut off tops of peppers; clean out seeds. Fill with rice mixture. Place in casserole.

3. Blend remaining 1 tablespoon olive oil into tomato puree. Pour over stuffed peppers.

4. Bake until peppers are tender, about 45 minutes. Serve hot.

ASPARAGUS ON TOAST WITH MUSHROOM SAUCE

¼ cup margarine
¼ cup whole-wheat flour
2 cups milk
½ pound mushrooms, sliced or chopped
1 teaspoon celery salt
Asparagus tips, lightly steamed
6 slices whole-wheat toast

1. Melt margarine in medium saucepan over low heat. Stir in flour and cook 3 minutes. Gradually increase heat to medium and stir in milk slowly, until smooth and thick, stirring constantly. Add mushrooms and simmer until tender. Season with celery salt.

2. Arrange asparagus tips on toast. Pour sauce over and serve.

STEAMED ASPARAGUS

Cut off lower parts of stalk as far down as they will snap. Place stalks of asparagus together and stand in deep covered kettle. Add water to come ¼ up stalks. Steam until tender, 5 minutes or less.

Serve with margarine, yogurt, or lemon juice. Season with celery salt, tarragon, or vegetable salt.

ARTICHOKES WITH YOGURT HERB SAUCE

2 cups yogurt
Juice of ½ lemon
½ teaspoon dill weed
½ teaspoon chopped parsley leaves
½ teaspoon sea salt
Pinch of garlic salt
Pinch of onion salt
Pinch of paprika
1 to 2 artichokes for each person, trimmed
Boiling water
Sea salt

Combine first 8 ingredients; chill.

1. Stand artichokes upright in wide, deep saucepan. Add 2 inches boiling water and a pinch of sea salt.

2. Cover and simmer until base of artichoke can be easily pierced with fork, about 30 minutes.

3. Lift out and drain well. Spread leaves gently, and remove fuzzy choke portion with a spoon.

Serve warm or cold with yogurt sauce.

WILD RICE AND MUSHROOMS

2 cups vegetable stock or water, boiling
1 cup raw wild rice
2 tablespoons oil
½ pound fresh mushrooms, sliced
5 tablespoons olive oil
2 cups finely chopped celery
1 onion, chopped
1 green pepper, chopped
½ cup tomato juice

1. Pour boiling stock or water over well-washed rice. Let stand overnight. The next day, liquid will be absorbed and rice ready to use.

2. Preheat oven to 350°F (175°C).

3. Heat 2 tablespoons oil in large skillet over medium heat. Add mushrooms and sauté until tender.

4. In another skillet, heat 5 tablespoons olive oil over medium heat. Add celery, onion, and pepper and sauté until tender. Combine with rice and mushrooms. Turn into oiled casserole and pour tomato juice over.

5. Bake mixture until liquid is absorbed. Serve hot.

BAKED BEANS AND TOMATOES

1 quart dried navy beans
3 cups chopped tomato
2 tablespoons honey
Vegetable salt, to taste

1. Soak beans overnight in enough water to cover.

2. Simmer until tender, about 1 hour. Drain.

3. Preheat oven to 250°F (120°C). Combine beans with all remaining ingredients in stoneware crock. Cover and bake 3 to 4 hours.

4. Remove cover and continue baking until top is browned. Serve hot.

PEAS WITH LEMON MINT SAUCE

3 cups fresh shelled peas
¼ cup margarine
2 tablespoons finely chopped fresh mint
1 tablespoon lemon juice
¼ teaspoon finely grated lemon peel

1. Steam peas in small amount of water until tender, about 10 to 15 minutes.

2. Stir in all remaining ingredients. Serve immediately.

BAKED MUSHROOMS

12 large mushrooms
¼ cup margarine
1 medium onion, chopped
1 teaspoon crushed garlic
1 green apple, chopped
¼ teaspoon each: thyme, parsley, celery seed, marjoram
1½ cups bread crumbs (dark rye is especially good)
¼ cup sunflower seeds
Sea salt, to taste

1. Preheat oven to 350°F (175°C).

2. Rinse and dry mushrooms. Remove and chop stems. Melt margarine in skillet over medium heat. Add onion, garlic, apple, herbs, and chopped mushroom stems and sauté until onion is tender.

3. Add bread crumbs and sunflower seeds and toss well. Add sea salt.

4. Place some stuffing in each mushroom cap, mounding it up on top.

5. Arrange in oiled casserole. Cover and bake 30 to 40 minutes. Serve hot.

MUSHROOM CASSEROLE

¼ cup oil
4 cups sliced mushrooms
1 onion, minced
¼ cup water
3 tablespoons brewer's yeast
1 teaspoon oregano
½ teaspoon rosemary

1. Preheat oven to 350°F (175°C).
Heat oil in large skillet over medium
heat. Add mushrooms and onion and
sauté until tender.

2. Add all remaining ingredients.
Turn into casserole. Cover.

3. Bake 20 minutes. Serve hot.

SPINACH FAR EAST

2 pounds spinach or beet tops,
   steamed
½ cup oil
1 onion, minced
½ cup sesame seeds
Juice of 1 lemon

Combine all ingredients. Chill before
serving.

STUFFED TOMATOES

1 cup cooked brown rice
1 onion, chopped
2 mushrooms, chopped
½ cup diced celery and tops,
   steamed
1 tablespoon oil
½ teaspoon thyme
½ teaspoon vegetable salt
6 large tomatoes, hollowed out

1. Preheat oven to 350°F (175°C).
Combine all ingredients except tomatoes. Spoon into tomatoes.

2. Arrange in oiled baking pan.

3. Bake 30 to 35 minutes. Serve hot.

BAKED TOMATOES

Several firm, large tomatoes, halved
   crosswise
Olive oil
Lemon juice
Tarragon
Chopped parsley leaves
Ground coriander
Vegetable salt

1. Preheat oven to 300°F (150°C).

2. Rub outsides of tomatoes with
olive oil. Arrange cut-side down
in shallow baking pan. Add small
amount of water and lemon juice to
bottom of pan. Sprinkle with tarragon, parsley, and coriander.

3. Bake 10 minutes, basting occasionally with pan liquid. Serve hot.

RATATOUILLE

1 medium-size eggplant, peeled
3 zucchini
2 to 3 tablespoons olive oil
3 firm tomatoes, coarsely chopped
1 large onion, sliced
3 cloves garlic, chopped
½ teaspoon oregano
Vegetable salt, to taste
Grated Parmesan cheese

1. Preheat oven to 300°F (150°C).

2. Cut eggplant and zucchini into
1½-inch cubes.

3. Heat olive oil in large skillet over
medium-high heat. Add eggplant and
zucchini and sauté until lightly
browned.

4. Remove from pan. Reduce heat and
add tomatoes, onion, garlic, oregano,
and vegetable salt. Simmer until
onion is limp.

5. Combine all ingredients in casserole. Cover and bake for 1 hour.
Serve hot or chilled.

SPINACH AND MUSHROOMS

2 pounds spinach
¼ cup margarine
1¼ pounds fresh mushrooms, sliced
½ onion, chopped
3 tablespoons yogurt
Vegetable salt, to taste
4 to 5 cups cooked brown rice

1. Rinse spinach well; do not dry. Steam in water clinging to leaves just until tender, about 3 minutes. Drain, reserving liquid. If necessary, add water to liquid to make ¼ cup.

2. Melt margarine in large skillet over medium heat. Add mushrooms and onion and sauté until tender.

3. Chop spinach. Add to mushroom mixture and cook 3 minutes.

4. Stir in spinach cooking liquid and yogurt.

5. Heat through and season with vegetable salt. Serve on rice.

GREEK SPINACH PIE (SPANAKOPITA)

1½ pounds feta cheese
Milk
2 pounds spinach, rinsed and stemmed
2 onions, chopped
3 tablespoons olive oil
1 pound creamed cottage cheese
4 eggs
¼ cup whole-wheat bread crumbs
½ pound filo pastry (available at a Mediterranean delicatessen)
½ cup (about) margarine, melted

1. Soak feta cheese overnight in enough milk to cover.

2. Steam spinach in water clinging to leaves just until beginning to wilt, about 3 minutes. Chop.

3. Heat oil in large skillet over medium heat. Add onions and sauté until transparent and slightly browned. Add spinach and cook for 1 minute.

4. Drain feta, discarding milk. Beat together feta, cottage cheese, and eggs. Stir in bread crumbs and spinach mixture.

5. Preheat oven to 350°F (175°C). Place 3 layers of filo pastry in 13 x 9-inch baking pan, brushing each sheet with melted margarine. Spoon on spinach mixture.

6. Cover filling with 2 to 3 more layers of filo, again brushing each with margarine. Tuck dough under to make neat edge. Brush top with margarine.

7. Bake 40 minutes. Let stand at room temperature 10 minutes before cutting.

DEEP-DISH SPINACH PIE

2 pounds raw spinach or beet tops, rinsed and cut into bite-size pieces
1 cup chopped green onions
½ cup chopped parsley leaves
2 tablespoons oil
½ teaspoon rosemary
⅓ teaspoon vegetable salt
Whole-wheat pastry for single crust (p. 161)
Cream

1. Preheat oven to 425°F (220°C). Combine spinach, green onions, parsley, oil, rosemary, and vegetable salt in large pot, place over medium heat and cook, stirring once or twice, just until mixture is reduced to half of original volume.

2. Turn into oiled casserole. Cover with pastry. Brush with cream.

3. Bake until pastry is browned, about 15 to 20 minutes. Serve hot or warm.

FILLED CABBAGE LEAVES

1 head Savoy cabbage
1½ cups steamed brown rice
2 onions, sliced and steamed
2 tablespoons whole-wheat cracker
  or bread crumbs
Minced parsley leaves
Thyme
Sage
3 cups tomato puree

1. Preheat oven to 350°F (175°C). Steam cabbage briefly. Separate leaves.

2. Mix rice, steamed onions, cracker crumbs, minced parsley, thyme, and sage.

3. Place a tablespoon of the mixture at the near end of each cabbage leaf, roll up part way, then turn in sides and continue rolling. Press gently between palms of hands.

4. Arrange stuffed cabbage leaves in casserole or roasting pan, edge side down. Pour tomato puree over.

5. Bake about 30 minutes. Serve hot.

MUSHROOM BROWN RICE

⅔ cup oil
1 cup chopped onions
2 cups sliced fresh mushrooms
6 cups cooked brown rice
Vegetable salt, to taste
¼ cup minced parsley leaves

1. Heat ⅓ cup oil in large skillet over medium heat. Add onions and sauté until tender. Remove with slotted spoon. Add mushrooms to skillet and sauté briefly.

2. Add remaining oil to cooked rice and toss lightly. Add mushrooms and onions. Season with vegetable salt. Serve hot, sprinkled with parsley.

CABBAGE AND CARROTS

3 tablespoons margarine or oil
1 small head cabbage, finely shredded
3 cups grated carrots
½ teaspoon dill weed
½ teaspoon caraway seeds
Lemon juice
Vegetable or sea salt

1. Heat oil in wok or skillet over medium heat. Add cabbage and carrots and stir-fry until crisp-tender.

2. Add herbs and cook until vegetables are tender. Stir in lemon juice and vegetable salt. Serve hot.

SPINACH QUICHE

Whole-wheat pastry for single
  9-inch pie crust (p. 161)
2 pounds fresh spinach, rinsed and
  stemmed
2 tablespoons chopped green onion
3 tablespoons margarine
1 cup yogurt
3 eggs, beaten
½ cup nonfat milk
½ teaspoon vegetable salt
½ teaspoon nutmeg
¼ cup grated Swiss cheese

1. Preheat oven to 375°F (190°C). Line 9-inch pie plate or tart pan with whole-wheat pastry.

2. Plunge spinach into large pot of boiling water for 1 minute. Drain very well; blot dry with paper towels. Chop.

3. Melt 2 tablespoons margarine in medium skillet over medium-high heat. Add green onion and spinach and cook until liquid is evaporated, about 2 to 3 minutes.

4. Combine yogurt, eggs, milk, and seasonings, and beat well. Blend in spinach mixture. Turn into crust. Sprinkle with cheese and dot with remaining margarine.

5. Bake until filling is set, about 25 minutes. Serve hot.

YELLOW CROOKNECK SQUASH

3 tablespoons olive oil or margarine
7 crookneck squash, sliced ½-inch
  thick
½ onion, chopped
Vegetable salt, to taste
Dash of fresh nutmeg
2 to 3 tablespoons water

1. Heat oil in large skillet over medium heat. Add squash, onion, vegetable salt, nutmeg, and water.

2. Cook until squash is tender. Serve hot.

SUMMER SQUASH

Squash, sliced
Egg, beaten
Whole-wheat bread or cracker
  crumbs

Preheat broiler. Dip squash slices in beaten egg, then in crumbs. Arrange on oiled pan. Broil until brown and tender, turning once. Serve hot.

CABBAGE WITH APPLES

1 head red cabbage, sliced
2 cups apple chunks
¼ cup oil
3 tablespoons apple juice
Cloves
Allspice
1 cup yogurt

Simmer cabbage, apples, oil, apple juice, and spices over low heat for 30 minutes, stirring occasionally. Add yogurt, and simmer 5 minutes more. Serve hot.

BAKED ONIONS

6 onions, preferably Bermuda
4 slices rye or whole-wheat toast,
  halved
Butter, softened
1 cup grated cheddar cheese
4 eggs, beaten
1 cup milk
3 tablespoons margarine

1. Cut onions in ½-inch slices and steam for 4 to 5 minutes.

2. Preheat oven to 350°F (175°C). Butter toast. Arrange in bottom of casserole. Place onions on top of toast. Cover with grated cheese.

3. Combine eggs and milk. Pour mixture over cheese. Dot with margarine.

4. Bake 30 minutes. Serve hot.

SCALLOPED BRUSSELS SPROUTS

1 pound Brussels sprouts
1½ cups chopped celery
3 tablespoons margarine
3 tablespoons whole-wheat flour
1½ cups scalded milk
1 cup whole-wheat bread crumbs
3 tablespoons margarine

1. Remove wilted leaves from Brussels sprouts. Steam until tender. Drain well.

2. Preheat oven to 400°F (205°C). Melt 3 tablespoons margarine in medium skillet over high heat. Add celery and cook 2 minutes.

3. Reduce heat to low and add whole-wheat flour. Slowly pour in scalded milk. Pour this mixture over sprouts.

4. Sprinkle with bread crumbs. Dot with remaining 3 tablespoons margarine.

5. Bake until crumbs are brown, about 10 to 15 minutes. Serve hot.

VEGETABLE STEW

2 tablespoons oil
2 onions, sliced
3 tomatoes, cut into wedges
1 cup cubed raw potatoes
1 cup sliced zucchini
½ cup grated carrots
½ cup grated parsnip
3 tablespoons brewer's yeast
3 tablespoons minced parsley leaves
1 sprig dill, minced

Heat oil in large skillet over medium heat. Add onion and sauté until transparent. Stir in remaining ingredients. Cover and simmer until tender.

BAKED SQUASH

3 small winter squash—acorn, butternut, etc.
½ cup sesame seeds
3 tablespoons honey
3 tablespoons oil or margarine
⅛ teaspoon ground mace

1. Preheat oven to 350°F (175°C). Cut squash in half. Remove seeds and membranes. Arrange in shallow pan. Add water to pan ¼-inch deep.

2. Blend all remaining ingredients. Spoon into cavities of squash.

3. Cover and bake until tender, about 1 hour, uncovering during the last 10 minutes of baking time to allow squash to brown. Serve hot.

BAKED GRATED ZUCCHINI

6 to 7 medium zucchini
¼ cup margarine
Parmesan cheese

1. Preheat oven to 400°F (205°C). Grate zucchini into oiled casserole approximately 13 x 8 x 2 inches. Dot with margarine and sprinkle with Parmesan cheese.

2. Bake until margarine is melted, about 10 to 15 minutes. Do not overcook; zucchini should be crisp-tender.

VEGETABLE SOYBEAN LOAF

1 cup grated raw carrots
1 cup cooked soybeans
1 cup grated raw beets
1 onion, grated
1 green pepper, minced
½ cup wheat germ
⅓ cup tomato juice
2 eggs
3 tablespoons soy flour
1 teaspoon oregano
1 teaspoon chopped parsley leaves
½ teaspoon vegetable salt
Cashew Gravy or Tamari Gravy
   (p. 147), optional

1. Preheat oven to 350°F (175°C). Blend all ingredients. Turn into oiled loaf pan.

2. Bake 1 hour. Serve hot. Can be served with Cashew or Tamari Gravy.

BAKED BEETS

1 bunch beets, trimmed
½ to 1 cup water
1 tablespoon olive oil

1. Preheat oven to 350°F (175°C). Scrub beets well. Arrange in baking dish. Add water and oil.

2. Cover and bake until tender, about 1½ hours. Serve whole or cubed.

SOYBEANS

4 cups sprouted soybeans
3 tablespoons soy oil
½ cup chopped onion
1 green pepper, chopped
¼ cup chopped olives

Sauce:
2 cups chopped tomatoes
2 tablespoons honey
Vegetable salt, to taste

1. Simmer soybeans in water to cover until tender, about 20 minutes.

2. Heat oil in large skillet over medium heat. Add onion, green pepper, and olives and cook until tender.

3. Stir in soybeans, tomatoes, honey and vegetable salt and heat through.

BROILED TOMATOES

1 cup whole-wheat bread crumbs
2 tablespoons chopped green onion
¼ teaspoon oregano
¼ teaspoon basil
¼ teaspoon vegetable salt
6 large tomatoes (unpeeled), cut into ¾-inch-thick slices
2 tablespoons olive oil
½ cup Parmesan cheese

1. Combine crumbs, green onion, herbs, and vegetable salt.

2. Dip tomato slices into crumb mixture. Pour oil into shallow pan; arrange slices in pan.

3. Place under broiler for about 2 minutes.

4. Sprinkle with Parmesan cheese, and return to broiler just until melted. Serve immediately.

GRATED TURNIPS

5 to 6 medium turnips
Vegetable salt, to taste
3 tablespoons margarine

1. Scrub and grate unpeeled turnips.

2. Preheat oven to 400°F (205°C). Spread turnips in oiled baking dish and season with vegetable salt. Dot with margarine. Bake until crisp-tender, 6 to 10 minutes. Serve hot.

STUFFED ZUCCHINI

2 or 3 large zucchini, partially steamed
¾ cup whole-wheat bread crumbs
2 tablespoons grated Parmesan cheese
¼ teaspoon oregano
¼ teaspoon sage
⅛ teaspoon marjoram
⅛ teaspoon rosemary
Additional grated Parmesan cheese

1. Preheat oven to 350°F (175°C). Scoop out centers of zucchini to make ¾ cup. Combine pulp with crumbs, 2 tablespoons Parmesan, and herbs.

2. Stuff zucchini shells with mixture. Bake 10 minutes. Sprinkle with Parmesan cheese and serve.

ZUCCHINI PANCAKES

4 to 5 medium zucchini, grated
3 eggs, whole
¼ cup whole-wheat flour
3 tablespoons grated Parmesan cheese
1 teaspoon minced parsley leaves
Pinch of garlic powder
Margarine

Combine all ingredients except margarine. Oil skillet or pancake griddle and heat to 375°F (190°C). Drop batter onto skillet and cook until brown, then turn and brown second side. Keep warm in 200°F (95°C) oven. Serve with dab of margarine.

BALKAN PILAF

¼ cup olive oil
2 large onions, chopped
2 cups raw brown rice
¼ cup chopped pignolias or almonds
¼ cup currants or raisins
4 cups stock
2 tomatoes, sliced
1 teaspoon sage
1 teaspoon chopped parsley leaves
½ teaspoon allspice
Vegetable salt, to taste

1. Heat oil in large skillet over medium heat. Add onions and sauté until transparent.

2. Stir in rice and nuts, and cook 5 minutes.

3. Add all remaining ingredients. Cover tightly and cook over very low heat until rice is tender and all liquid is absorbed, about 30 to 40 minutes. (A burner pad is helpful.) Serve hot.

BAKED POTATOES IN JACKETS

Baking potatoes, uniform in size
Vegetable oil
Margarine

1. Preheat oven to 425°F (220°C). Scrub potatoes well and dry. Brush with oil to keep skins tender and moist. Cut off tip ends.

2. Bake potatoes until tender, about 50 minutes. Serve with margarine. (Remember that the skins contain important nutrients and should be eaten whenever possible.)

PARSNIPS IN CIDER

8 parsnips, peeled
⅔ cup apple cider
6 tablespoons margarine
⅓ cup firmly packed brown sugar

1. Preheat oven to 400°F (205°C). Cut parsnips in fourths lengthwise. Simmer in water to cover until almost tender.

2. Arrange parsnips in baking dish. Mix remaining ingredients and spread over parsnips.

3. Bake 20 minutes, basting occasionally. Serve hot.

SAUCY CUCUMBERS

2 tablespoons oil
2 tablespoons sliced green onion
¼ cup yogurt
¼ cup lemon juice
2 tablespoons honey
4 cucumbers, sliced

1. Heat oil in large skillet over medium heat. Add green onion and sauté until transparent. Let cool.

2. Mix yogurt, lemon juice, and honey and blend with cucumbers and onion. Chill before serving.

BAKED ASPARAGUS

Steamed asparagus (reserve cooking water for sauce)
1 cup bread crumbs
Celery salt
Paprika
1 tablespoon margarine
Grated cheese

1. Preheat oven to 300°F (150°C). Cut steamed asparagus into 1-inch lengths.

2. In oiled baking dish, alternate layers of asparagus with bread crumbs, celery salt, and paprika between each layer. Over all pour several tablespoons water left after steaming asparagus. Dot top with margarine.

3. Bake 20 minutes. Just before removing from oven, sprinkle top thickly with grated cheese. Let melt. Serve hot.

MARINARA SAUCE

¼ cup olive oil
½ eggplant, diced
1 onion, chopped
2 stalks celery, chopped
½ bell pepper, chopped
1 clove garlic, minced
1 4-ounce can tomato paste (without preservatives, or make your own)
1 cup water
6 to 8 tomatoes, chopped
½ teaspoon oregano
½ teaspoon basil
Parmesan cheese

1. Heat olive oil in large skillet over medium heat. Add eggplant, onion, celery, pepper, and garlic, and sauté until tender.

2. Dilute tomato paste with water. Add to skillet with tomatoes and herbs.

3. Simmer about 45 minutes. Serve over artichoke spaghetti or whole-wheat noodles. Sprinkle with Parmesan cheese.

CHEESE SOUFFLÉ

¼ cup margarine
¼ cup whole-wheat flour
1 cup milk
1½ cups grated cheddar cheese
½ teaspoon thyme
6 eggs, separated
Dash of vegetable salt

1. Preheat oven to 350°F (175°C). Melt margarine in medium saucepan over low heat. Add flour and stir 3 minutes. Gradually add milk and cheese, stirring constantly.

2. Add thyme and cook until smooth and thick. Remove from heat.

3. Beat in egg yolks and vegetable salt.

4. Beat egg whites in large bowl until stiff. Fold into cheese mixture. Pour into oiled deep soufflé or deep baking dish.

5. Bake until puffed and golden, about 1 hour. Serve immediately.

BEETS AND TOPS

4 beets with tops
1 tablespoon margarine
Vegetable salt, to taste
2 tablespoons lemon juice

1. Wash beets and tops well. Cut away tops; chop coarsely. Steam in water clinging to leaves until tender.

2. Grate beets and add to tops with margarine and vegetable salt.

3. Simmer 5 minutes. Stir in lemon juice and serve.

BAKED POTATO DISH

Potatoes
Margarine
Onion, minced
Parsley leaves, minced

1. Preheat oven to 375°F (190°C). Slice raw potatoes thinly. Arrange layer in shallow baking dish. Dot with margarine. Sprinkle generously with onion and parsley.

2. Add another layer of sliced potatoes. Sprinkle with onion and parsley. Dot with margarine.

3. Cover and bake until potatoes are tender, about 45 minutes. Remove cover and continue baking until browned.

BLENDER SPINACH SOUFFLÉ

1 pound spinach, stemmed and steamed
1 cup stock or water
4 eggs, separated
¼ cup grated cheese
3 tablespoons whole-wheat flour
3 tablespoons brewer's yeast
¼ teaspoon vegetable salt

1. Preheat oven to 375°F (190°C). Combine all ingredients except egg whites in blender and blend until smooth.

2. Beat egg whites in large bowl until stiff. Fold into spinach mixture. Turn into oiled soufflé dish or oiled individual custard cups.

3. Bake until puffed and golden, about 35 to 40 minutes for large souffle, about 30 minutes for individual custard cups. Serve immediately.

RISOTTO

¼ cup oil
1 onion, chopped
1 clove garlic, minced
1 cup raw brown rice
2 cups vegetable stock or water
3 tablespoons minced parsley leaves
½ teaspoon rosemary
Pinch of saffron
½ cup grated cheddar cheese

1. Heat oil in large skillet over medium heat. Add onion, garlic, and rice and sauté until golden.

2. Pour in ½ of stock. Sprinkle in parsley, rosemary, and saffron, and cook over low heat, adding more stock as liquid is absorbed.

3. When rice is tender and all liquid is absorbed, sprinkle in cheese and stir until just melted. Serve hot.

NUT LOAF

3 cups whole-wheat bread crumbs
1½ cups chopped nuts
1 cup finely chopped celery
1 cup tomato juice
½ cup finely chopped onion
¼ cup chopped parsley leaves
3 tablespoons oil
Vegetable salt, to taste

1. Preheat oven to 350°F (175°C). Combine all ingredients and blend well.

2. Pack into oiled loaf pan and bake 45 minutes.

Serve with Tamari Gravy (p. 147).

SPROUTED WHEAT BURGERS

2 cups steamed millet
2 cups sprouted wheat
½ cup sunflower seeds
½ cup bread crumbs
¼ cup minced onion
2 tablespoons peanut butter
2 tablespoons oil
2 tablespoons soy sauce
½ teaspoon thyme
½ teaspoon sea salt

Combine all ingredients and blend well. Form into patties and brown on both sides in skillet or on griddle.

Serve with Cashew Gravy (p. 147).

POTATOES AU GRATIN

Potatoes (new potatoes are especially good), steamed and diced
Grated cheese
Margarine
Whole-wheat bread crumbs
Milk

1. Preheat oven to 375°F (190°C). Place layer of potatoes in shallow baking dish. Sprinkle generously with grated cheese. Dot with margarine. Repeat until baking dish is almost filled.

2. Top with layer of whole-wheat bread crumbs. Dot with margarine. Add milk just to top of potatoes.

3. Bake until crumbs are browned, about 30 minutes. Let stand at room temperature 10 minutes before serving.

STUFFED POTATOES

Potatoes, as uniform in size as
  possible
Margarine
Onion, finely minced
Yogurt
Parsley leaves, minced

1. Preheat oven to 425°F (220°C).
Bake potatoes until tender, about
45 minutes to 1 hour.

2. Halve lengthwise. Scoop out
insides. Mash with margarine, finely
minced onion, and yogurt, to taste,
beating until smooth. Replace in
shells.

3. Return to oven and bake until
browned.

4. Sprinkle with minced parsley
and add a dot of margarine. Serve
hot.

POTATO PANCAKES

5 potatoes, scrubbed
1 onion, grated
¼ cup chopped parsley leaves
1 egg
Vegetable salt, to taste
Oil or margarine

1. Grate potatoes finely. Add onion,
parsley, egg, and vegetable salt and
mix well.

2. Heat oil in heavy skillet. Drop
batter by large spoonfuls onto
skillet. Brown on one side, then
turn and brown second side. Serve
hot.

OLIVE-STUFFED PEPPERS

6 medium-size bell peppers
2 cups whole-wheat bread crumbs
1 cup of seeded and chopped ripe
  olives
1 cup grated cheese
1 cup milk
1 small onion, finely chopped
Margarine

1. Preheat oven to 350°F (175°C). Cut
off tops of peppers; clean out seeds.

2. Combine all remaining ingredients,
except margarine. Spoon into peppers. Place small piece of margarine
on top of each.

3. Arrange in oiled baking dish. Bake
until peppers are tender, about 45
minutes. Serve hot.

MACARONI AND CHEESE

2 cups vegetable macaroni noodles
  or shell macaroni
1½ cups milk
½ cup nonfat dry milk powder
1 cup grated cheddar cheese
⅔ cup whole-wheat bread crumbs
  (optional)
¼ cup margarine (optional)

1. Bring large pot of water to rapid
boil over high heat. Slowly add
macaroni. Boil until almost tender.

2. Preheat oven to 400°F (205°C).
Remove macaroni from heat and
drain. Blend in milk, powdered
milk, and cheese.

3. Pour into oiled baking dish. If
desired, sprinkle with crumb topping made by mixing bread crumbs
with margarine.

4. Bake until bubbly and browned,
about 15 minutes. Serve hot.

BAKED EGGPLANT WITH TOMATO

1 large eggplant
Tomato, raw or cooked
Onion, chopped
Green pepper, chopped
Olive Oil

1. Preheat oven to 400°F (205°C). Bake eggplant until tender, about 30 minutes. (Do not turn oven off.)

2. Cut into slices about 1 inch thick. Arrange in baking dish, alternating layers of sliced eggplant and slices of raw (or cooked) tomato. Season each tomato layer with chopped onion and green pepper. Dribble on oil by tablespoonfuls.

3. Bake 20 to 30 minutes. Serve hot from baking dish.

SWEET POTATOES BAKED WITH HONEY

6 sweet potatoes or yams, cooked
    and halved lengthwise
½ cup honey
¼ cup oil
Juice of 1 lemon
Pinch of mace

1. Preheat oven to 350°F (175°C). Arrange sweet potatoes in oiled casserole.

2. Mix remaining ingredients and pour over sweet potatoes.

3. Bake about 30 minutes, basting occasionally. Serve hot.

CASHEW GRAVY

2 cups water
½ cup raw cashews
2 tablespoons arrowroot
2 tablespoons soy sauce
2 tablespoons oil
2 teaspoons onion powder

1. Combine all ingredients in blender and puree until smooth.

2. Transfer to small saucepan and cook over medium heat, stirring, until thickened. Serve hot.

TAMARI GRAVY

3 tablespoons sesame oil
½ cup chopped mushrooms
¼ cup chopped onion
1½ cups water
2 tablespoons tamari (soy sauce)
1 tablespoon arrowroot

1. Heat oil in medium skillet over medium heat. Add mushrooms and onion and sauté until tender.

2. Combine water, soy sauce, and arrowroot and stir until smooth. Slowly stir into mushrooms and onion. Let simmer a few minutes, until thickened. Serve hot.

BREADS AND MUFFINS

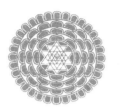

WHEAT GERM MUFFINS

1 cup milk
1 egg, beaten
3 tablespoons honey
3 tablespoons oil
1 cup wheat germ
1 cup whole-wheat flour
4 teaspoons baking powder
½ teaspoon sea salt

1. Preheat oven to 400°F (205°C). Oil muffin pans or line with paper muffin cups.

2. Combine milk, egg, honey, and oil and blend well. Stir in wheat germ.

3. Sift together flour, baking powder, and salt. Add to wheat germ mixture and stir just until combined; do not overmix.

4. Fill prepared muffin pans halfway with batter. Bake until browned, about 20 minutes.

Makes about 20 2-inch muffins.

WHOLE-WHEAT BREAD

½ cup molasses
¼ cup margarine or oil
4 teaspoons sea salt
2 cups warm milk (105°F to 115°F; 40° to 45°C)
2 cups warm water
2 tablespoons dry yeast
10 to 12 cups whole-wheat flour

1. Stir molasses, margarine, and salt into milk in large bowl. Add water and yeast.

2. Add half of flour and beat until smooth. Knead in remaining flour. Knead well and place in very large oiled bowl, turning dough to coat entire surface with oil.

3. Cover with towel and let rise in warm draft-free area until doubled in volume. Punch down and let double again.

4. Form into 4 loaves. Place in oiled 9 x 5-inch loaf pans and let rise until dough reaches tops of pans.

5. Preheat oven to 350°F (175°C).

6. Bake until loaves sound hollow when tapped, about 1 hour. Turn out onto racks to cool before slicing.

Makes 4 9 x 5-inch loaves.

CORNBREAD

2 cups cornmeal
2 teaspoons baking powder
½ teaspoon sea salt
1 cup milk
1 egg, beaten
2 tablespoons oil
1 tablespoon honey

1. Preheat oven to 400°F (205°C). Sift together cornmeal, baking powder, and salt.

2. Add milk, egg, oil, and honey and stir to blend.

3. Pour into oiled 8-inch square pan. Bake until golden, about 30 minutes.

WHOLE-WHEAT MUFFINS

2 cups whole-wheat flour
3 tablespoons baking powder
¼ teaspoon sea salt
1 cup milk
1 egg, beaten
3 tablespoons oil
¼ cup honey
½ cup raisins

1. Preheat oven to 375°F (190°C). Oil muffin pans or line with paper muffin cups.

2. Stir together flour, baking powder, and salt.

3. Combine milk, egg, oil, and honey and blend well. Stir into flour mixture with raisins. (Do not beat; batter should be lumpy.) Fill prepared muffin pans ⅔ full with batter. Bake until browned, about 20 minutes.

Makes about 20 2-inch muffins.

SUNFLOWER BREAD

3 tablespoons honey
1 envelope yeast
⅓ cup warm water (105° to 115°F; 40° to 45°C)
2 tablespoons margarine
1 teaspoon sea salt
1¼ cups boiling water
1¾ cups whole-wheat flour
1¾ cups sunflower seed meal (process sunflower seeds in blender until fine)
⅓ cup raisins

1. Stir honey and yeast into warm water and let stand until foamy, about 5 minutes.

2. Add margarine and salt to boiling water and let cool to lukewarm.

3. Combine flour, meal, and raisins with the yeast mixture, in large bowl. Turn out onto floured board and knead well.

4. Place in very large oiled bowl, turning to coat entire surface with oil. Cover with towel and let rise in warm draft-free area until doubled in volume.

5. Punch down. Place in oiled 9 x 5-inch loaf pan and let rise until dough reaches top of pan.

6. Preheat oven to 350°F (175°C).

7. Bake until bread sounds hollow when tapped, about 60 minutes. Turn out onto rack to cool before slicing.

Makes 1 9 x 5-inch loaf.

BANANA BREAD

¼ cup oil or ½ cup margarine
½ cup honey or ⅔ cup raw sugar
3 to 4 ripe bananas, mashed
3 eggs, beaten
2 cups whole-wheat pastry flour
1 tablespoon baking powder
¼ teaspoon sea salt
⅔ cup milk
⅓ cup chopped pecans or raisins
½ teaspoon vanilla

1. Preheat oven to 350°F (175°C). Cream oil and sugar in large bowl. Add bananas and eggs and beat well.

2. Stir dry ingredients together and blend into banana mixture. Add milk, nuts or raisins, and vanilla.

3. Pour batter into oiled 8 x 10-inch pan. Bake at 350°F until tester inserted in center comes out clean, about 50 minutes.

Makes 1 8 x 10-inch loaf.

CEREALS

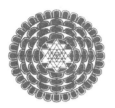

ENZYME VITAMIN CEREAL

7 tablespoons wheat germ
2 tablespoons raw sugar
4 teaspoons brewer's yeast
1 tablespoon chia seeds
1 tablespoon sesame seeds
1 tablespoon rice polishings
2 teaspoons sunflower seed meal
Milk, fruit, or orange juice (garnish)

Combine all ingredients. Serve with milk, fruit, or orange juice.

Makes about ¾ cup.

SWISS BREAKFAST

6 apples, grated
1 cup fresh berries, if available
½ cup raw oats, soaked overnight in 1 cup water
½ cup yogurt
¼ cup ground hazelnuts or almonds
Juice of 2 lemons
3 tablespoons honey
Yogurt and berries (garnish)

Combine all ingredients and blend well. Top with dollop of yogurt and a fresh berry or two.

Makes 8 to 9 cups.

GOOD MORNING!

1 cup water
½ cup raisins
½ cup hulled sunflower seeds
Juice of 1 lemon
3 bananas, sliced
2 apples, grated
½ cup wheat germ
1 cup yogurt

1. Combine water, raisins, sunflower seeds, and lemon juice and let soak 1 hour.

2. Mix in bananas, apples, and wheat germ. Top with yogurt and serve.

Makes 6 to 7 cups.

CRUNCHY GRAIN CEREAL

½ cup honey
¼ cup molasses
3 tablespoons oil
3 cups rolled oats
1 cup puffed millet
½ cup unsweetened grated coconut
½ cup sesame seeds
¼ teaspoon sea salt

1. Preheat oven to 250°F (120°C). Combine honey, molasses, and oil in medium saucepan and heat through.

2. Combine with all remaining ingredients in roasting pan and mix well.

3. Bake until golden, stirring occasionally. Let cool before storing airtight.

Makes 5 to 6 cups.

WHEAT CEREAL

1 quart water
2 cups cracked wheat
½ cup raisins

Combine all ingredients and soak overnight.

Makes about 4 cups.

VACUUM-BOTTLE COOKED CEREAL

1 quart water
⅔ cup whole wheat
⅓ cup whole oats
⅓ cup barley
1 tablespoon hulled sunflower seeds

1. In the morning, combine all ingredients and let soak 8 to 12 hours.

2. Drain water into large measuring cup. Add more water to total 3 cups.

3. Bring water to boil in large saucepan. Add soaked ingredients and boil 1 minute.

4. Pour into 1-quart vacuum bottle and turn on side overnight.

5. Cereal will be ready to eat the next morning.

Makes about 1 quart.

STEAMED BROWN RICE

2 cups water
1 cup raw brown rice
Milk or yogurt
Fruit
Honey (optional)

Bring water to boil in medium saucepan. Sprinkle in rice. Cover and cook gently until all liquid is absorbed, about 30 to 40 minutes. Serve with milk or yogurt and fruit. Sweeten with honey if desired.

Makes about 2 cups.

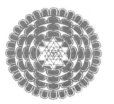

BUCKWHEAT PANCAKES

1 cup warm milk (105° to 115°F; 40° to 45°C)
1 cup yogurt
2 tablespoons margarine or butter, melted
1½ teaspoons dry yeast
1½ cups buckwheat flour
1 teaspoon baking soda
1 teaspoon sea salt

1. Combine milk, yogurt, margarine, and yeast and blend well. Let stand in a warm place overnight.

2. In the morning, stir in flour, baking soda, and salt. Bake on lightly oiled griddle, flipping pancakes when edges appear dry and bubbles appear in center.

Makes about 18 2½-inch pancakes.

RICE WAFFLES

2 cups brown rice flour
5 teaspoons baking powder
⅛ teaspoon sea salt
2 cups water
3 tablespoons sesame oil
1 tablespoon honey

1. Sift together flour, baking powder, and salt.

2. Blend water, oil, and honey. Stir into flour mixture.

3. Bake in waffle iron.

Makes about 6 waffles.

WHOLE-WHEAT EGGLESS WAFFLE BATTER

2 cups whole-wheat pastry flour
2 tablespoons soy flour
2½ teaspoons baking powder
½ teaspoon cinnamon
½ teaspoon sea salt
2½ cups milk
2 tablespoons soy oil
1 cup blueberries (optional)

1. Sift together dry ingredients. Slowly add milk and oil, stirring gently until nearly smooth. Add blueberries if desired.

2. Bake in waffle iron or on *lightly* oiled griddle over medium heat. Test griddle by dropping one drop of water on it. If water steams away rapidly, griddle is ready. For pancakes, flip when edges appear dry and bubbles appear in center.

Makes about 6 waffles.

FRUIT DESSERTS

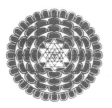

BAKED PEARS

6 pears, unpeeled
¼ cup honey
¼ cup lemon juice
2 tablespoons oil or melted
    margarine

1. Preheat oven to 350°F (175°C).
Halve pears lengthwise; core. Arrange
in oiled baking dish, cut sides up.

2. Blend honey, lemon juice, and oil
and pour over pears.

3. Bake until tender, about 15 minutes.
Serve warm or cold.

Makes 6 servings.

FRUIT DESSERT SUPREME

1 cup sliced bananas
1 cup sliced oranges
1 cup sliced pineapple
1 cup sliced pears
1 cup yogurt
½ cup pecans or walnuts
1 tablespoon honey
Nutmeg, to taste

1. Combine all fruits in large bowl
and toss gently.

2. Blend yogurt, nuts, honey and nutmeg and stir into fruit. Chill at least 1
hour before serving.

Makes 6 servings.

CRISPY TOPPED APPLES

6 to 8 apples, preferably pippin
½ cup raisins
¼ teaspoon nutmeg
¼ teaspoon cinnamon
½ cup apple juice
1 cup raw sugar
½ cup whole-wheat pastry flour
¼ cup sesame seeds
3 tablespoons margarine

1. Preheat oven to 375°F (190°C).
Rinse, core, and slice apples. Peel if
they have been sprayed; otherwise
leave unpeeled.

2. Combine apples and raisins in
oiled casserole. Sprinkle on spices
and pour cider over.

3. Work remaining ingredients together with fingers until crumbly.
Spread over apples as topping.

4. Bake uncovered until apples are
tender, about 45 minutes. Serve warm.

Makes 6 to 8 servings.

COOKED DRIED FRUIT COMPOTE

Place selected dried fruit in saucepan with tight-fitting lid. Add small
amount of water, place over low heat
and steam 45 minutes, adding more
water if necessary.

UNCOOKED DRIED FRUIT COMPOTE

Soak selected dried fruits in enough apple or orange juice to cover overnight.

Yogurt makes an excellent topping, if desired.

BLENDER APPLESAUCE

3 to 4 crisp apples, preferably
    Jonathans or Gravensteins
¼ to ½ cup apple juice
1 tablespoon lemon juice
¼ cup honey

1. Rinse, core, and slice apples. Peel if they have been sprayed; otherwise leave unpeeled.

2. Combine apple juice, lemon juice and honey in blender. Add apples until container is ⅓ full.

3. Puree at medium-high speed, adding remainder of apple slices. Chill and serve.

Makes 2 to 3 cups.

STEWED APPLES

1½ pounds firm apples
¾ cup water
3 tablespoons raw sugar or honey
1 tablespoon lemon juice

1. Rinse, core, and cut apples into ½-inch slices. Peel if they have been sprayed; otherwise leave unpeeled.

2. Combine apples and water in saucepan and simmer until barely tender. Add sugar or honey and lemon juice. Simmer 1 minute more. Let cool and serve with liquid.

Makes 6 servings.

BAKED APPLES

4 or more large apples, preferably
    Rome Beauty
½ cup boiling water
Cinnamon, to taste
Nutmeg, to taste
Cloves, to taste
½ cup raw sugar

1. Preheat oven to 450°F (230°C). Rinse and core apples. Peel upper ¼ of apples; arrange peeled side down in boiling water in large saucepan. Simmer until tender, about 10 minutes.

2. Arrange apples peeled side up in baking dish. Sprinkle with spices and sugar.

3. Bake until browned, about 10 minutes. Serve warm.

STEWED PEARS

3 pears
1 cup fresh orange juice
¼ cup honey or 2 tablespoons raw
    sugar
1 teaspoon grated orange rind

1. Rinse pears and halve lengthwise. Core. Combine pears and orange juice in saucepan and simmer until tender.

2. Remove pears using slotted spoon. Add honey or sugar and grated rind to juice.

3. Simmer syrup 3 minutes longer. Pour over pears. Chill thoroughly before serving.

Makes 6 servings.

BERRY YOGURT

3 cups strawberries, blueberries, or
    raspberries
1 cup plain yogurt
¼ cup honey

Combine ¼ cup of the berries with remaining ingredients in blender and puree until smooth. Spoon over remaining berries. Chill before serving.

Makes 6 servings.

PRUNE WHIP

2 cups prunes
Spring water or apple juice
¼ cup pignolias or almonds
Honey, to taste.

1. Soak prunes overnight in just enough spring water or apple juice to cover.

2. Remove pits. Combine prunes and soaking liquid in blender and puree until smooth. Stir in nuts. Sweeten with honey if desired.

Makes 6 servings.

BLUEBERRIES IN YOGURT

2 cups blueberries (fresh if possible; otherwise, frozen)
1 cup yogurt
3 tablespoons honey

Mix all ingredients and chill. (If desired, strawberries or peaches may be used in place of blueberries.)

Makes 4 to 6 servings.

BAKED RHUBARB

1½ pounds rhubarb, cut into 1-inch pieces
Boiling water
1½ cups raisins
⅓ cup pineapple, orange, or apple juice
1 cup fresh berries
Mace

1. Leach out oxalic acid from rhubarb by pouring boiling water over; let stand 10 minutes, then drain well.

2. Preheat oven to 350°F (175°C). Combine rhubarb, raisins, and fruit juice and place in oiled casserole.

3. Cover and bake until tender, about 25 minutes. Serve with garnish of fresh berries. Sprinkle with mace.

Makes 6 servings.

BROILED BANANAS

Bananas
Margarine
Raw sugar
Mace

Preheat broiler. Halve bananas lengthwise. Dot with margarine; sprinkle with raw sugar and mace.

Broil until lightly browned. Serve hot.

FRUIT CUP

6 to 8 apricots, pitted and chopped
1 to 2 oranges, diced
1 banana, sliced
½ cup fresh or frozen berries
Honey

Combine all fruits and toss gently. Sweeten to taste with honey. Chill before serving.

Makes 4 to 6 servings.

FIG AMBROSIA

3 large oranges
1 pound fresh figs, sliced
½ cup orange juice
5 tablespoons grated coconut
½ teaspoon grated orange peel

Peel oranges. Separate segments, removing membranes and seeds. Combine oranges with all remaining ingredients and toss gently. Chill before serving.

Makes 6 servings.

FRUIT JUICE GELATIN

½ cup vegetable gelatin (agar-agar)
1½ cups water
2 cups fruit juice of your choice
¼ cup honey

1. Combine agar-agar and water in medium saucepan and let stand until softened, 5 to 10 minutes.

2. Place over low heat and simmer until agar-agar is dissolved.

3. Add fruit juice. Sweeten with honey if desired. Allow to set; it will jell rapidly. Chill before serving.

Makes 6 servings.

BANANA-LEMON SAUCE

2 ripe bananas
½ cup honey
3 to 4 ounces cream cheese, cut in cubes
¼ to ⅓ cup raisins
Juice of 1 lemon
Grated rind of ½ lemon
Plain cake or pudding

Combine bananas, honey, cheese, raisins, lemon juice, and rind in blender and puree until smooth. Serve over plain cake or pudding.

Makes about 2 cups.

RAW CRANBERRY SAUCE

1 cup fresh cranberries
1 apple, cored and quartered
½ ripe banana
Juice of 1 orange
1 tablespoon grated orange rind
Honey, to taste

Combine all ingredients in blender and puree until smooth.

Makes 1 to 1½ cups.

PUDDINGS AND CUSTARDS

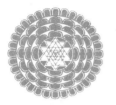

UNCOOKED HOLIDAY PUDDING

2 cups ground almonds
2 crisp apples, grated
2 carrots, grated
1 cup minced raisins and/or currants
4 ounces bread crumbs
¼ cup orange juice
2 pieces candied ginger, minced
2 tablespoons candied citrus peel
2 teaspoons grated orange rind
Dash of mace

1. Combine all ingredients and blend well.

2. Press into oiled pudding mold or large bowl. Cover with plate; top with weight. Refrigerate at least overnight, preferably several days.

Makes 6 servings.

POLYNESIAN COCONUT PUDDING

5 tablespoons honey
3 tablespoons arrowroot
½ cup grated coconut
2 cups coconut milk
Strawberries or oranges

1. Combine honey, arrowroot, and coconut in medium saucepan. Gradually stir in coconut milk. Place over medium heat and cook until thickened; do not boil.

2. Pour into individual dishes. Let cool, then chill. Top with sliced strawberries or oranges.

Makes 4 to 6 servings.

COTTAGE CHEESE CUSTARD

2 cups (1 pound) cottage cheese
2 eggs
¼ cup honey
2 tablespoons raisins
Cinnamon, to taste

Preheat oven to 325°F (165°C). Combine all ingredients and blend well. Turn into oiled 1½-quart baking dish. Bake until set, about 20 to 25 minutes. Serve warm or cooled.

Makes 4 to 6 servings.

EGGLESS RICE PUDDING

4½ cups milk
½ cup raw brown rice
½ cup raw sugar
½ cup raisins
½ teaspoon vanilla
Nutmeg

Preheat oven to 300°F (150°C). Combine all ingredients except nutmeg and pour into oiled baking dish. Sprinkle with nutmeg. Bake 3 hours, stirring occasionally. Serve warm or cooled.

Makes 4 to 6 servings.

DATE RICE PUDDING

1 quart milk
½ cup raw sugar or honey
¼ cup uncooked brown rice
¼ teaspoon sea salt
¼ teaspoon nutmeg
1 cup chopped dates

1. Preheat oven to 300°F (150°C). Mix all ingredients except dates. Turn into oiled 2-quart casserole.

2. Bake 1 hour, stirring occasionally.

3. Stir in dates and bake 2 hours more. Serve warm or cooled.

Makes 4 servings.

RICE CUSTARD

2 cups milk
½ cup raisins
⅓ cup cooked brown rice
⅓ cup honey
2 eggs
1½ teaspoons vanilla

1. Preheat oven to 325°F (165°C). Mix all ingredients. Turn into oiled custard cups or baking dish.

2. Bake until knife inserted in center comes out clean, about 1 hour. Serve warm or cooled.

Makes 4 servings.

APRICOT CUSTARD

2 cups milk
½ cup unsulfured dried apricots
⅓ cup honey
3 eggs

1. Preheat oven to 350°F (175°C). Combine all ingredients in blender and puree at highest speed, scraping down sides of container as necessary. Blend about 3 minutes.

2. Pour into oiled custard cups. Set cups in pan of boiling water.

3. Bake until knife inserted in center comes out clean, about 45 minutes. Cool before serving.

Makes 4 to 6 servings.

ICE CREAM AND SHERBET

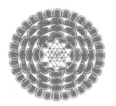

HONEY-CARROT ICE CREAM

3 cups fresh carrot juice
1 cup raw milk
1 cup raw whipping cream
¾ cup honey
2 teaspoons vanilla

Mix all ingredients well and process in ice cream freezer according to manufacturer's instructions.

If ice cream freezer is unavailable, ice cream can be frozen in refrigerator freezer compartment as follows: Pour into shallow container and freeze until ice crystals have formed ¾ inch deep around container. Remove and beat well. Return to freezer until mushy but not quite solid. Remove and beat again. Replace in freezer until firm.

Makes about 2 quarts.

BANANA-ORANGE SHERBET

3 ripe bananas
2 cups yogurt
1 cup orange juice

Mash bananas and beat in remaining ingredients. Freeze in freezer compartment of refrigerator, beating twice during freezing process as described for Honey-Carrot Ice Cream.

Makes about 1 quart.

PASTRIES

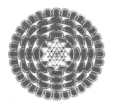

APPLESAUCE CAKE

¾ cup honey
⅓ cup margarine, softened
2 eggs, beaten
1½ cups whole-wheat flour
½ cup soy flour
¼ teaspoon mace
¼ teaspoon cloves
¼ teaspoon cinnamon
⅛ teaspoon sea salt
¾ cup applesauce
½ cup raisins

1. Preheat oven to 350°F (175°C). Cream honey and margarine in large bowl. Add eggs and beat well.

2. Sift dry ingredients together and add to honey mixture. Add applesauce and raisins and beat well.

3. Turn batter into greased 9-inch square pan. Bake until tester inserted in center comes out clean, about 45 minutes. Cool before serving.

Makes 1 9-inch square cake.

CANADIAN DATE CAKE

1½ cups chopped dates
½ cup water
2 tablespoons raw sugar
1 cup sifted whole-wheat pastry flour
⅛ teaspoon sea salt
1 cup margarine, softened
1 cup raw sugar
1 teaspoon vanilla
2 cups rolled oats

1. For filling, combine dates, water, and sugar in medium saucepan and simmer gently until dates are very tender; stir frequently to keep mixture from scorching.

2. Remove from heat and mash with fork. Set aside while preparing crumb mixture.

3. Preheat oven to 325°F (165°C). Sift flour and salt together. Cream margarine, sugar, and vanilla. Stir in flour mixture and oats.

4. Divide in half and pat one half on bottom of 8-inch square cake pan. Spread with date filling. Top with remaining crumb mixture.

5. Bake until tester inserted in center comes out clean, about 1½ hours. Serve warm or cooled.

Makes 1 8-inch square cake.

UNBAKED CHEESECAKE

2½ cups cream cheese, softened
1¼ cups yogurt
¼ cup honey
1 teaspoon vanilla
9-inch unbaked crumb crust

1. Combine cream cheese and yogurt in large bowl and beat well. Blend in honey and vanilla.

2. Turn mixture into crust and refrigerate until firm. Serve chilled.

Makes 1 9-inch round cake.

COCONUT PIE CRUST

1 cup shredded coconut
½ cup wheat germ
¼ cup whole-wheat flour
2 tablespoons margarine, softened
2 tablespoons honey

Preheat oven to 400°F (205°C). Combine all ingredients and blend well. Press into pie pan. Bake until golden, about 5 to 7 minutes. Cool before filling.

Makes 1 9-inch crust.

WHOLE-WHEAT PIE CRUST

1½ cups whole-wheat pastry flour
½ teaspoon sea salt
½ cup wheat germ
⅔ cup margarine, well chilled
¼ cup ice water

1. Preheat oven to 425°F (220°C). Sift flour and salt into large mixing bowl. Stir in wheat germ. Cut margarine into flour with pastry blender (mixture should resemble pebbles). Sprinkle in water and mix lightly with fork; do not overmix or crust will be tough.

2. Roll out half of dough on floured board into 10½-inch circle. Drape gently around rolling pin; unroll into 9-inch pie pan with ¾-inch overlap. Tuck overlap under and flute edge. If shell is to be prebaked, prick bottom with fork. Bake until lightly colored, about 8 to 10 minutes.

NOTE: For double crust, turn filling into unbaked shell. Roll out dough for top crust, place on filling, and tuck under overlap. Flute edge. Cut slits in crust for steam to escape.

Makes 2 9-inch pie shells or 1 double 9-inch crust.

CAROB CAKE

1⅔ cups raw sugar
½ cup margarine, softened
2 eggs
½ cup water
½ cup carob powder
2½ cups sifted whole-wheat pastry flour
½ teaspoon baking soda
½ teaspoon sea salt
⅓ cup yogurt
⅓ cup milk
Banana-Lemon Sauce (page 156)

1. Preheat oven to 350°F (175°C). Cream sugar and margarine in large bowl. Add eggs and beat well.

2. Combine water and carob powder and stir until smooth. Blend into sugar mixture.

3. Sift dry ingredients together twice. Add ½ dry ingredients to carob mixture, then add yogurt and milk. Mix well and add remaining dry ingredients.

4. Turn batter into greased 13 x 9-inch pan. Bake until tester inserted in center comes out clean, about 30 to 35 minutes. When cool, cut in slices and serve with Banana-Lemon Sauce.

Makes 1 13 x 9-inch cake.

CARROT CAKE

5 carrots
1 cup water
7 eggs, separated
2 cups raw sugar
1 tablespoon grated orange rind
3 cups grated almonds

1. Preheat oven to 325° F (165°C). Cook carrots in the water until tender. Drain (save water for soup stock). Mash carrots and let cool.

2. Beat egg yolks and sugar until mixture forms ribbons when beaters are lifted. Add the carrots, orange rind, and almonds and blend well.

3. Beat egg whites until stiff; fold into carrot mixture.

4. Turn batter into greased 9-inch springform pan.

5. Bake until toothpick inserted in center comes out clean, about 45 minutes. Cool before serving.

Makes 1 9-inch round cake.

CAROB MACAROONS

1 cup margarine
1 cup honey
2 eggs, beaten
2 cups sifted whole-wheat flour
1 teaspoon baking powder
1 teaspoon baking soda
½ cup carob powder
½ teaspoon sea salt
1 cup rolled oats
1 cup grated coconut
½ teaspoon almond extract

1. Preheat oven to 350°F (175°C).
Cream margarine. Add honey gradually and beat well.

2. Beat in eggs.

3. Sift together flour, baking powder, baking soda, carob, and salt. Add to creamed mixture with oats, coconut, and almond extract. Mix well.

4. Drop by teaspoons onto oiled cookie sheet.

5. Bake until edges begin to brown, about 12 to 15 minutes. Transfer to racks to cool.

Makes 5 to 6 dozen.

ZUCCHINI CUPCAKES

2 eggs
¾ cup safflower or corn oil
½ cup raw sugar
½ cup honey
1½ cups finely grated zucchini
1½ cups whole-wheat pastry flour
½ cup carob powder
1 teaspoon cinnamon
¾ teaspoon baking powder
½ teaspoon baking soda
½ teaspoon sea salt
¼ teaspoon cloves
¼ teaspoon cardamom
¼ teaspoon anise seed
½ cup raisins
Cream Cheese Frosting (optional)

1. Preheat oven to 350°F (175°C).
Beat eggs until fluffy. Add oil, sugar, and honey, and beat well. Stir in zucchini.

2. Sift together dry ingredients, and add to liquid mixture with raisins. Mix well.

3. Fill greased muffin tins ½ full.

4. Bake until tester inserted in center comes out clean, about 20 minutes. (If you would rather have a cake, turn into greased 9 x 12-inch pan and bake at 350°F (175°C) for about 40 minutes.)

5. Cool. Frost with Cream Cheese Frosting if desired.

Makes 15 to 18.

CREAM CHEESE FROSTING

8 ounces cream cheese, softened
2 tablespoons margarine, softened
¼ cup honey

Cream cheese and margarine well.
Beat in honey a little at a time.

Makes about 1¼ cups.

CHEESE CAKE

1 pound cream cheese, softened
½ cup honey
1 tablespoon arrowroot
¼ cup orange juice
1 teaspoon vanilla
1 teaspoon lemon juice
1 teaspoon grated lemon rind
9-inch unbaked crumb crust

1. Preheat oven to 350°F (175°C).
Combine cream cheese and honey and beat well.

2. Dissolve arrowroot in orange juice.
Add to cream cheese mixture with vanilla, lemon juice, and lemon rind and beat well.

3. Turn mixture into crust. Bake until filling is set, about 20 minutes.
Cool before serving.

Makes 1 9-inch round cake.

CAROB BROWNIES

¾ cup whole-wheat pastry flour
1 teaspoon baking powder
½ teaspoon sea salt
½ cup melted margarine
½ cup honey
2 eggs, beaten
½ cup carob powder
1 tablespoon melted margarine
1 cup chopped nuts or hulled
    sunflower seeds
1 teaspoon vanilla

1. Preheat oven to 350°F (175°C).
Sift together flour, baking powder,
and salt.

2. Beat melted margarine, honey,
and eggs. Add flour mixture.

3. Combine carob powder with 1
tablespoon melted margarine. Add
to flour mixture with nuts and vanilla.
Mix well. Spread in greased 9-inch
square pan.

4. Bake until firm, about 30 minutes.
Do not overbake.

Makes 1 9-inch square pan.

PUMPKIN PIE

2 cups milk
1¾ cups mashed cooked pumpkin
    or squash
⅔ cup raw sugar
3 eggs, beaten
1 teaspoon cinnamon
1 teaspoon vanilla
1 teaspoon sea salt
¼ teaspoon ginger
¼ teaspoon cloves
¼ teaspoon mace
9-inch unbaked pie shell

1. Preheat oven to 450°F (230°C).
Mix all filling ingredients and blend
well. Turn into pie shell.

2. Bake 10 minutes. Reduce heat
to 325°F (165°C) and bake until
knife inserted halfway between center and edge of pie comes out clean,
about 40 to 50 minutes. Cool before
serving.

Makes 1 9-inch pie.

CRUMB CRUST

16 graham crackers (stone-ground
    graham crackers are available in
    health food stores)
⅓ cup margarine, softened
3 tablespoons raw sugar
¼ teaspoon cinnamon

1. Preheat oven to 400°F (205°C).
Crush graham crackers with rolling
pin or in blender to make fine
crumbs. Mix crumbs with all remaining ingredients.

2. Press firmly onto sides and bottom
of 9-inch pie pan.

3. Bake until golden, about 6 minutes.
Cool before filling.

Makes 1 9-inch crust.

GINGERSNAPS

4 cups whole wheat flour
1⅓ cups molasses
½ cup melted margarine
1 tablespoon ginger
1 tablespoon cinammon
2 teaspoons baking soda
½ teaspoon cloves
½ teaspoon sea salt

1. Preheat oven to 350°F (175°C).
Combine all ingredients in large bowl
and blend well.

2. Drop by teaspoons onto greased
cookie sheet. Flatten with bottom of
oiled glass.

3. Bake until golden, about 15 minutes. Transfer to racks to cool.

Makes about 12 dozen.

SESAME SEED COOKIES

1 cup raw sugar
½ cup oil or margarine
1 egg, beaten
1¼ cups rolled oats
¾ cup sesame seeds
½ cup raisins
2 tablespoons milk
1¼ cup whole-wheat pastry flour
½ teaspoon nutmeg

1. Preheat oven to 375°F (190°C). Cream sugar and oil in large bowl. Add egg and beat well.

2. Mix oats, sesame seeds, raisins, and milk. Stir into sugar mixture.

3. Sift together flour and nutmeg. Add, and mix well.

4. Drop dough by teaspoons onto oiled cookie sheet. Flatten with bottom of oiled glass or fork.

5. Bake until brown, about 10 minutes. Transfer to racks to cool. Makes about 4 dozen.

BLACKSTRAP COOKIES

2½ cups sifted whole-wheat pastry flour
2 teaspoons baking powder
1 teaspoon ginger
½ cup wheat germ
⅔ cup blackstrap molasses
⅓ cup honey
½ cup margarine or oil

1. Preheat oven to 350°F (175°C). Sift together flour, baking powder, and ginger. Stir in wheat germ.

2. Heat molasses and honey in large saucepan until just warm enough to melt margarine; add margarine. Blend in dry ingredients.

3. Chill for 1 hour.

4. Roll dough out on floured board and cut out shapes with floured cookie cutter. Transfer to lightly greased cookie sheet.

5. Bake 10 to 12 minutes. Transfer to racks to cool.

Makes 5 to 6 dozen 2-inch cookies.

OATMEAL COOKIES

4 cups rolled oats
2 cups whole-wheat flour
1 cup honey
¾ cup oil
¼ cup apple or orange juice
1 teaspoon vanilla
½ teaspoon cinnamon
½ teaspoon nutmeg

1. Preheat oven to 350°F (175°C). Combine all ingredients in large bowl and blend well.

2. Drop by teaspoons onto greased cookie sheet.

3. Bake until golden, about 15 minutes. Transfer to racks to cool.

Makes about 100.

CANDIES AND OTHER SWEET TREATS

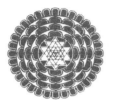

UNBAKED CAROB COOKIES

2 cups pitted dates
1 cup raisins
½ cup chopped pecans or pignolias
Carob powder

1. Put dates, raisins, and nuts through food grinder.

2. Mix in carob powder until mixture will not hold any more and dough is stiff enough to roll. Roll out and cut into bars.

3. Place in direct sunlight for 1 day to dry.

SESAME CANDY

1 cup tahini
½ cup creamed honey
¼ cup chopped pignolias
¼ cup carob powder
3 tablespoons rice polishings
2 tablespoons grated coconut
2 tablespoons vanilla
Toasted sesame seeds
Finely grated coconut

1. Combine tahini, honey, pignolias, carob, rice polishings, 2 tablespoons coconut, and vanilla and knead well.

2. Shape mixture into balls; roll in sesame seeds and coat with coconut. Chill until firm.

Makes about 1¼ pounds.

DATE CANDY

3 cups pitted dates
½ cup raisins
1 cup chopped pecans or other nuts
Ground nuts
Finely grated coconut

1. Put dates and raisins through food grinder.

2. Mix in chopped nuts. Knead with hands until well blended. Form into 1-inch-diameter log. Roll in ground nuts and/or coconut.

3. Wrap in waxed paper and chill until firm, several hours or overnight. Cut into slices.

STUFFED DATES

Pitted dates make be stuffed with
the following:
Cashew butter
Blanched almonds
Hulled sunflower seeds
Pecans
Sesame Candy (page 165)

Serve plain or roll in finely grated
coconut. Can be stored in an airtight
container and kept in refrigerator
several weeks.

APRICOT LEATHER

3 to 5 pounds ripe apricots
¼ cup raw sugar for each cup of
   puree

1. Wash, peel, and pit apricots. Mash
or puree in blender. Stir in raw sugar.

2. Transfer to large saucepan and
place over low heat until mixture
comes to boil. Boil for 2 minutes.
Pour into large shallow pan or dish
and spread paste to 1/16-inch thickness.
Cover with cheesecloth.

3. Set outside in full sunshine for a
few days until paste has dried to a
tough, leatherlike consistency. Cut
into large squares and roll into cylin-
ders. Wrap in waxed paper. Keeps
well.

Makes 2 to 3 pounds.

TAHINI CANDY

1 cup nonfat dry milk powder
½ cup crystallized or creamed honey
⅓ cup carob powder
2 tablespoons tahini
¼ teaspoon vanilla
Finely grated coconut or carob powder (optional)

1. Combine all ingredients except
coconut or carob and knead well.

2. Form into roll. Chill until firm;
slice. Slices can be coated with coconut or carob powder.

Makes about ⅓ pound.

MOLASSES-WHEAT GERM CANDY

2½ cups toasted wheat germ
1 cup almond butter
1 cup nonfat dry milk powder
1 cup raisins
½ cup blackstrap molasses
½ cup honey

Combine all ingredients and knead
well. Press into oiled 8-inch square
pan and cut into 1-inch squares.

Makes 64 pieces.

SESAME-FRUIT CANDY

1 pound dried apricots
1 pound pitted dates
½ cup raisins or prunes
½ cup dried figs
1 tablespoon sesame or soy oil
½ cup plus 6 tablespoons sesame
   seeds
2 tablespoons creamed honey

1. Put fruits through food mill.

2. Toast seeds as follows: Place ½
cup oil in skillet, add sesame seeds,
cover, and shake a few minutes over
medium heat. (Seeds pop like pop-
corn as they brown.) Peek in to see
when seeds are golden brown. Set
aside 6 tablespoons seeds.

3. Mix remaining seeds with fruits
and honey. Shape mixture into balls
and roll in reserved seeds. Chill until
firm.

Makes about 2 pounds.

PART 4

PHILOSOPHY AND MEDITATION

PRINCIPLES

I

WHAT WE ARE NOT

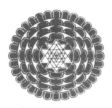

The basic premise of Yoga philosophy is that we see ourselves as something other than we really are. We look at ourselves in a type of distorted mirror—like the kind you find in an amusement park—and because the mirror is imperfect, the image of ourselves and the way in which we see the world is reflected to us as similarly distorted. We laugh when we see ourselves in this distorted form because we are able to make the comparison between the way we know we really look and the way the mirror has changed our appearance. And yet, it is exactly this distortion that we accept in our everyday lives: We mistake the distortion for the real and unquestioningly accept what is false for what is true. And because all of our problems—anxieties, frustrations, fears, and sense of unfulfillment—are the inevitable consequence of not understanding that we accept the false for the true, the philosophy and meditation of Yoga is concerned with pointing out this distinction, with providing the means for the student to discern the way in which he has lost sight of his true nature and how his Reality can be rediscovered.

First, let us be clear on the meaning of *reality* as it pertains to our Yogic study. What is born and dies, and is subject to continual change between birth and death, is transient—changing, transforming, and vanishing. What vanishes, what we perceive at one time and then at some point no longer perceive, is like a mirage. A mirage is unreal. Inherent in all that is unreal is illusion and frustration. In Yoga, the unreality of what is constantly changing and vanishing is contrasted with that which is eternal, never-changing, without qualities, and beyond duality. This eternal principle, which is your true nature, is designated as Self, God, or Reality; and Self-Realization means that you have recognized your true nature, you have recovered what was misplaced.

The body, a temporary sheath in which you find yourself contained, cannot be considered real in the way we have described reality. Your body is changing each moment; it is dying. Since your true nature is that of eternal Self, you are not the body. The fact that the body's senses, nervous system, brain, and so forth perform their various functions and interpret to you experiences —pain, hunger, gratification— does not mean that your true Reality is that of the body. The body dies, but the Self does not die. Self has no birth and no death. Understand that you are Self and you will find that everything is instantly transformed. The way in which you act in the world and your relationships with the people and objects of the world assume a totally different perspective because you recognize that you are not in the world but the world is *flowing through you*. You are not a separate self, seeking to gratify the ego's desires, but you are One with All.

The unenlightened person identifies with and limits himself to a body, making it the focal point of existence. He maneuvers this alien body through an alien world seeking happiness, fulfillment, and peace. But this quest has no possibility of success. The unenlightened person is like the thirsty man on the desert who, each time he sees a mirage of water, believes it will quench his thirst. He reaches out to drink and the water vanishes. In the same way, each time you feel you are on the verge of finally achieving your goals by having arranged things in the external world as you want them to be, you find you cannot maintain these conditions, that your goals begin to slip away. Why? Because everything you deal with in the external world is constantly changing and you can never freeze conditions as you would like. The wise men speak of life that is lived in this type of quest—identifying with a body and seeking fulfillment in what appears to be an external world—as incessant suffering, disappointment, restlessness, and frustration. With a little thought you will agree that whatever fulfillment, peace, and happiness you think you have experienced has been transient. Your fulfillment is incomplete because however fulfilled you imagine yourself to be, you soon find yourself needing additional fulfillment. Whatever peace of mind you have known soon degenerates into new turmoil.

Because permanent fulfillment and happiness are inherent in Self and is man's true nature, it is sought by everyone. People engage in every imaginable activity to experience what they believe constitutes happiness. But because change is the nature of the mind, the world that the mind perceives is an entity in which all things are forever changing. Therefore, happiness that is gained through activity or acquisition cannot remain. Those conditions and qualities that today make something attractive and desirable, something worth the devotion of all your attention and energy are changing; since the conditions and qualities are impermanent, the attraction it has for you cannot endure. Therefore, the desires for new possessions, new situations, new activities are endless, and these endless desires result in endless pursuits and endless frustrations. But as often as a man's desires are thwarted, he continues to believe that he can eventually capture whatever it is he is seeking. He is very slow to realize that his situation is like someone who attempts to pick up a handful of water. The water runs through his fingers. He does not recognize that his mind, the entity that is sending him on the endless wild-goose chase after happiness in the world, is the same entity that is making it impossible for him to realize such happiness. Let us examine this situation.

The mind, a thinking machine that is not unlike a computer, appropriates unlimited power, and falsely acting as an omnipotent guide, convinces you that if you will follow its directions, it will lead you to fulfillment. Because, since the time of your birth, and in countless previous lifetimes, you have been conditioned to believe that happiness, success, and fulfillment are the true goals of life and are attainable, you permit yourself to fall under the spell of the mind and be hypnotized by its endless promises. The fact that you, and all with whom you come in contact, never achieve the happiness that has been promised, does not deter you from continuing the activities that are dictated by your mind. When, time and time again, you fail to achieve the ultimate peace, happiness, and fulfillment that you seek, you are convinced by your mind, the computer, that your failure is due to circumstances, bad luck, destiny, incompetency, and so forth. You fail to place the blame where it lies: You do not recognize that what the mind has promised, it cannot deliver! It is an entity that computes, that has the capacity to deal only in statistics and qualities, regardless of how profound, complex, or abstract these statistics and qualities may be. As such, it is totally incapable of providing the fulfillment it promises. Its ingenious treachery lies in the fact that it is able to convince you again and again that it *can* provide what you seek.

Early in life you learn to depend on your mind to make all things possible and to place your unqualified trust in it. Indeed, you worship it. "The mind of man!" you exclaim. "What is beyond its ability?" Your trust in it is continually reinforced by all people with whom you come in contact. Everyone is seeking happiness and gratification, and everyone is relying on his mind to furnish the necessary directions. So, of course, you go along unquestioningly. No one says, "Hey, wait just a moment. What if all these things we're doing and acquiring and thinking don't lead to what we *really* want and *really* need? What if our minds have been deceiving us all the time?" This, of course, is a difficult conclusion to reach, because you feel that if you can't trust your own mind, who can you trust? But if you begin to question the faith you have placed in the mind, if you begin to feed questions into the mind-computer regarding the position of omnipotence and guidance it has assumed, you may get some very revealing readouts.

When Dorothy confronted the Wizard of Oz and called his bluff, his facade collapsed. He admitted that it was through promises and intimidation that he kept the population of Oz in line. Like the donkey who pursues the carrot that is held in front of his head—and in the process is made to keep moving—you may find that you too are made to perpetually engage in the computer games of the mind, because it has con-

vinced you that without your total dependence upon it, you cannot function and you certainly cannot know fulfillment.

Is it not extraordinary that you know almost nothing about your thinking process and yet, without question, you allow this process to govern your life? You do not know from where thoughts come or to where they go. You say, "I am thinking," but what you really mean is that you are aware of a thought that is present now, at this moment. You did not say, "Now I will have this thought." You did not summon forth that thought. It simply appeared, and it will be succeeded by another thought that will appear and disappear, and so on endlessly. But because it is you who are aware of this succession of thoughts, you refer to them as "my thoughts." You give them your full attention and act upon them as they direct you to do. But are they really *your* thoughts? Is your true nature, your Self, composed of these things called thoughts? You probably imagine that thoughts come from somewhere within you, perhaps what is designated as a subconscious, and they travel through your mind like a train through a tunnel. But you have no actual awareness of such a process. It is only an idea. All you

know is that a thought is present at this moment, and that is all you ever know about thoughts and what you think of as your "mind."

It is this elusive mind, together with the emotions, that compose the ego. The ego is the illusion that gives rise to the feeling of an individual self, which we refer to as "I" and "mine." My self appears to be separate from the world and separate from all of the other selves that appear to populate this external world. Once you have this sense of a separate self, your Oneness assumes the illusion of parts and you become threatened by these other selves, as well as by the multiple forces of the world. Having what you believe to be an ego that is subject to losses, adversities, injuries, and even extinction, the business of your life becomes the protection of the ego. The major activities of your existence are involved with such protection. At all times you want the ego to be safe from everything that might diminish it. You try not only to protect it, but at the same time to have it grow and reinforce its reality by the continual gratification of its desires.

Perhaps you can begin to see the absurdity of this situation: You are involved with an illusionary ego, a nonexistent "I" that is seeking to be permanently fulfilled in a world that it populates with its own fantasies. By imprisoning you in this situation, the ego effectively diverts you from calling its bluff, from discovering that it is nothing more than a shadow, a phantom, and thereby from regaining your true identity, which is Self. You are never other than Self, but this fact is obscured by the dream of the ego. Your original, true, pure, spotless, immutable nature is that of Happiness. You have no need to seek it. Only discard all that is of the ego and Happiness emerges as the sun, which is always out but may be obscured by the clouds, and is seen only when the clouds dissolve.

This Happiness is not the opposite of unhappiness. Temporal happiness comes and goes and you cannot hold it, try as you will. Temporal happiness begets the need for additional happiness and you pursue it everywhere. But your chase after happiness causes you much unhappiness. The situation is like that of the man who forgets he has put a precious gem in his pocket. Thinking he has lost it, he travels far and wide to regain it. Because the gem is always with him, he could terminate his unhappy quest at any time by putting his hand in his pocket. In the same way, hav-ing forgotten that Self, Happiness, Bliss is your true nature, you seek it elsewhere. But it is always in your pocket. You may look into a creek and say that the water is muddy. The water is never muddy. The soil has mixed with it and if the soil is filtered, the purity of the water is again seen. The shadow of the ego is superimposed upon Self and obscures it, as the tip of your little finger, by being held in the right position, can obscure the immensity of the sun. Remove these impediments and the Self, eternal and ever-present, emerges. The practice of Yoga is for the purpose of removing the superimposition of the ego, dissolving it in Self, as a wave that is formed from the ocean but is never apart from it has a momentary identity as a wave and then merges with and dissolves into the ocean. Although referring to that formation as a "wave," no one suggests that it is apart from the ocean. In the same way, no matter how we may erroneously think of ourselves in terms of shapes, forms, and individual selves, we can never be apart from Self.

Now, lest the mind convey the image of Self as an entity in which all things are *contained*, it is necessary to state that *nothing exists in Self*. There is nothing apart from Self that exists *within* it and that can go *out* from it. Self IS. Do the rays of the sun exist *in* the sun? No, the rays *are* the sun; the rays never go out from the sun, although we may speak of them as if they did. The nature of the mind is to divide, split, separate, dissect, diversify, make many of the One, present the many as apart from the One and, ultimately, have the many entirely obscure the One. In this way, the parts are made to appear as "real" parts and the One is concealed. But regardless of how the rays of the sun are examined, analyzed, broken into a spectrum, or transformed into energy, they remain the sun—not an aspect of the sun, or something that is emanating from the sun, but the *sun itself*. Similarly, regardless of how the mind examines, analyzes, divides, and transforms in order to depict the phenomenal world to you in a particular way, All Is Self. You Are Self. Nothing is other than, or apart from Self.

2

THE WORLD WITHIN THE MIND

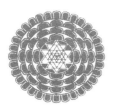

In the Yoga scriptures it is explained that the word "Self" is used to indicate that the Absolute we are attempting to describe is Self-luminous. It shines by Its own light that has no beginning and no end. It is dependent upon nothing and is not affected by, nor does it react to, any occurrence in the phenomenal world. It is further characterized as having the qualities of Bliss and Knowledge. That is, when you manifest as that which you truly Are, the experience is one of unqualified Joy and direct (not relative) Knowledge. We have already described Bliss and Happiness. Let us now look into the nature of Knowledge.

We must distinguish between relative knowledge (small k) and Knowing. The mind never Knows anything. It can only know *about* things, and knowing *about* things is relative knowledge. All relative knowledge has been described by one *Guru* as "learned ignorance." The mind can never wholly and completely encompass something and Know its nature, because it can never merge with anything. Its function is to analyze, distinguish, examine, investigate, assess, evaluate. To function in this manner necessitates a subject-object relationship with everything it perceives. That

is, no matter how subtle or abstract the examination, the mind remains outside or apart from that which it examines. But in order to grasp the *essence* of something it is necessary to merge, to accomplish Yoga with it. The mind and senses can inform you of the shape, odor, color, texture, and taste of an apple. But these are only qualities, things *about* the apple. What is the essence, the true nature of the apple? To know this, one must *become* the apple. In becoming the apple, the subject-object condition is dissolved, and because the subject-object relationship is a condition of the mind, the mind is also absorbed in the merger. Terminating the subject-object duality, in which you remain forever on the outside so that you are a separate self, always observing but never *experiencing* what is apart from you, can be achieved through the classical meditation techniques that are presented in the Meditation section.

The mind is concerned with knowledge about things that are alien to itself. Its nature is to flow *outward* and examine what is external. Therefore, what the mind appears not to know is endless because it is continuously projecting an infinite universe. It would have you believe that you are

perceiving an external universe, an entity absolutely real and apart from you, and that the ingenuity and resourcefulness of other minds in various fields of research will eventually know the "secrets" of the universe. But the mind can never, in the ultimate sense, Know. It can manufacture a universe and then appear to go in search of the "mysteries" of that universe. It can even convince you that it is on the verge of important discoveries about itself. But what it does is gather facts and statistics that it analyzes, evaluates, and investigates. It advances theories, which it then proceeds to modify on a monthly or yearly basis as new evidence is "discovered." It speaks with authority on man's problems and it abstracts concepts of spirit and God. But it is really whistling in the dark about all of this. It can never Know, because it remains in a perpetual subject-object relationship with that which it pretends it wants to know.

Each time the mind solves a problem, it is certain to fabricate a multitude of additional problems. It convinces you that your problems are external to yourself and that it serves you as a faithful servant by instructing you in the way to solve your problems. But, like the unscrupulous exterminator who, as he exterminates, plants the eggs for new insects so that you will require his additional services, the mind is always at work generating many more problems than it is solving, so that it ensures its position. The Truth is that all problems are created by the mind-computer and there can be no end to your problems unless there is an end to the problem maker. The ego manufactures the problems because that is its nature, that is what it does. As Self, or Awareness, which is what you Are, there can be no problems.

Our objective is not to permanently suppress thoughts or eliminate the process of thinking. We recognize that thoughts are necessary to assist us in performing what we perceive to be our duties in life. But they are not our Reality. They arise from the ego-shadow and they have no power to affect our true nature. When we thoroughly understand their nature, thoughts become our servants and can do us no harm. But when we act upon them as if we were an ego, then they rule our lives and do great damage, for they involve us in a futile chase after fulfillment and prevent us from being what we truly Are.

The method for achieving Self-Realization involves eliminating, transcending, dissolving the ego. These are different words all indicating the same process. Because the ego, although an illusion, is a formidable opponent, it is extremely helpful to have an intellectual comprehension of how it operates. In any confrontation—and the manner in which we must deal with the ego may certainly be thought of as a confrontation, if not an actual battle—it is wise to know as much as possible about that which you are confronting. We have already gone into some depth as to the way in which the ego (the mind and emotions) obscures one's recognition of Self. But there are other powerful illusions it manifests that must be examined. It is, of course, the mind that is doing the examining, but as you read these words the mind may be shaken a bit, sufficiently to cause a chink in its armor so that the light of Self may penetrate. The Wizard of Oz employed various contraptions to project his illusions. What are the devices of the ego?

Your Reality, Self, can be imagined as the screen in a movie theater. Onto this screen are projected the various scenes of a motion picture. A multitude of situations are depicted: disasters, adventure, romance, intrigue, and you become emotionally and mentally involved with each. You identify with the various characters and are swept into their situations. You cry and laugh with them, you share their triumphs and failures, and if the film is particularly gripping, you may find yourself emotionally and mentally drained at the conclusion. But then the film ends, the house lights are turned on, and you see that the screen is exactly as it was before the film began. It has not been burned by the fire, or drenched by the flood, or ripped by the tornado that was depicted. In a similar way, the ego projects or superimposes a world onto the screen of your Reality. You become hypnotized with this world and go through the multitude of physical, mental, and emotional involvements that are associated with "living." Just as while you watched the movie you accepted the situations as real and were swept into the scenes, so do you regard the world as real and act accordingly. And like the screen, your Reality is never affected by anything that is superimposed upon it. Your true nature cannot be touched.

The characters projected on the screen appear to move, and from the moment we consent to be hypnotized by this movement we do not question it. We know that the people and events we are witnessing are not really on the screen, but for the purposes of deriving experiences from the film there is a tacit agreement we make with ourselves to accept the illusion as real. Not only are the people and events not on the screen, but they are not really moving. It is the film—a series of still photographs—travelling through the projector that conveys the illusion of movement. In a similar way, not only is the world that is projected by the ego-mind an illusion, but it has no movement. The events that are witnessed as occurring in the world are actually the projections and movements of the mind. The world does not move, *it is the mind that moves*. From the moment we become hypnotized by movement in the world, we no longer question it. We may question the type of movement and how we are to involve ourselves with this movement, but we do not question the reality of movement and the events themselves. If, while viewing the film, it should suddenly break or become stuck on one frame, you are jarred out of the illusion. The movement has stopped and you are forced into recognition of the illusion you have been accepting as real.

It is this very situation that we attempt to deliberately induce by our Yoga practice. We attempt to stop the movement of the film (mind) so that the illusion of the reality of the world and the reality of all that appears to be occurring therein is exposed. We literally jar you out of your hypnotic state. When the film breaks in the theater, you do not need to search for the screen. It immediately appears because it has always been there. Indeed, among the elements of characters, plot, events, and movement, the screen is the only reality. Similarly, when you are released from the hypnosis of your mind and the infinite illusions it projects, you need not search for Self. It emerges the moment the mind is stopped, and you recognize that the characters, plots, events, and movements of the world have, all along, been superimposed upon it. This is Self-Realization. Stopping the movements of the mind is a basic objective of Yoga practice. Patanjali, a great *Guru* who lived in India several thousand years ago and who is credited with synthesizing the Yogic practices into an eight-step structure, stated, "Stop the movements of the mind and you will experience Yoga (Realization)."

The practice of *Hatha* Yoga is a great aid in this process. The mind is united to the energies of the body and as these energies are quieted and then redirected, the mind is restrained, and can also be redirected from its outward projections to an inward investigation. This is why it is highly effective to practice meditation immediately following your *Hatha* sessions. *Hatha* prepares you for productive meditation by effecting a profound quieting of the mind and senses. This quieting and redirecting of the mind is the primary objective of *Hatha* Yoga. The high level of health and fitness that result from the practice are actually by-products.

Let us suppose that you took a primitive person to see his first film. Imagine his terror as the speeding locomotive races ever closer. You would be hard put to convince him that his fears were groundless because there was really no locomotive, only moving pictures. Think, also, of his disbelief when you told him that the pictures weren't coming from the screen, but were being projected from behind him! The workings of this magic would have to be explained and demonstrated in some detail before he would understand the nature of the illusion. And so it is that we experience fear and anxiety from the pictures that we, ourselves, project. To understand that our fears are groundless and that we project our illusions out of ignorance requires explanation. This explanation is accomplished through investigation and must be undertaken by the student because, ultimately, the student must explain the illusion to himself. As has been previously pointed out, the type of Knowledge that is involved is beyond the mind, but the mind is used for the preliminary work. The mind must be lured into such an investigation because it is suspicious of anything that it perceives as being beyond its analytical capabilities. If it senses a threat of exposure, it will put up fierce resistance and this resistance usually takes the form of attempting to convince you that nothing is to be gained through meditation, that it's all just a waste of time, time that would be far more productively spent in your pursuit of its fantasies. Most people quickly accept this argument.

But there are those who, upon hearing or reading this doctrine, *will* be attracted to the necessary practices. Why are there people who almost immediately, or after some little time, are seriously drawn to the practice, while others dismiss the teachings as without personal value, having no relevance to their lives? The Yogi informs us that the former group is composed of those who, either intuitively or deliberately, are searching for enlightenment. He describes them as having "awakened from the dream of the ego" and contrasts them with those who remain asleep, hypnotized by the empty promises of the mind and, like blind men, grope about in the darkness for gratification. The awakened person has begun to suspect that something is wrong, that the way in which he has sought happiness is not working. He is looking for another route—he has become a "seeker."

Having once awakened, a seeker may intermittently nap, but cannot return to his undisturbed sleep. Deep stirrings, welcome or unwelcome, will prod this person. He will experience occasional flashes of illumination; the light comes and goes and the inner guidance is not yet clear. So, although he is drawn to and is guided by his inner Reality, he is also still subject to the delusions of the sleeping man. Therefore, the seeker has the feeling of being pulled in two directions simultaneously: toward the light and toward the world. This pulling frequently generates a profound conflict that is a natural development in the overall process. Eventually, the seeker understands that he is in the position of a traveler plodding along a path that, at its beginning, is dimly lighted. He trudges forth, encountering obstacles and frequently stumbling. He may briefly rest, may even temporarily reverse course. But ultimately will find the strength to resume his forward movement.

This traveler is involved in the greatest adventure possible and understands that time and progress are not factors in the quest; no obstacles can dissuade him. The irony is that reaching his destination, the seeker discovers he has been there all along; he has never left home! That is, returning to one's Reality the ego finds that it has never been apart from that Reality, as the wave can never be apart from the ocean. But there is no short-cutting this procedure. The ego must be led back to its source, as a stray horse is led back to the corral. The horse had gone to graze in a distant pasture, forgetting that his hay was waiting for him in his stall.

It is important to understand that the journey is not accomplished in steady, progressive, forward steps. We can illustrate this with a circle. The circumference represents the world of the ego-mind and the center represents Reality. As the seeker travels around the circumference, along with the sleeping man, his practice enables him, unlike the sleeper, to make intermittent jumps into the center where his Reality is experienced. But because clarity of vision is not yet fully developed and the outward pull of the mind is strong, his stay in the center is temporary. The seeker is pulled back to the circumference and this in-and-out movement composes the "conflict" indicated above. However, each time he or she returns to the circumference the seeker carries with him greater conviction about Reality and more insight into the illusion. His stay on the circumference becomes increasingly shorter, and those in the center, longer. When the jump into the center becomes permanent, when the ego is absorbed into Reality, the Realized person understands that the circumference has never existed and that there is only the center. From the circumference, the center—Reality—can be imagined, but once in the center there is no trace of a circumference. All is only the center. The ego-mind can conjure up a concept of Reality, but the *actual* Reality cannot contain an ego. In Yoga literature, there is the quotation of the king who attained Self-Realization. In wonder, he exclaimed, "The pretender (ego) who has been robbing me of my kingdom has vanished!"

REINCARNATION: THE CONSEQUENCE OF DESIRE

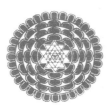

What causes a sleeping person to awaken? Are there a series of specific events that precipitate an awakening? In this connection, it is appropriate to examine the doctrine of *karma*. *Karma* is defined as "cause and effect." However gross or subtle, and however immediate or delayed, every action has a reaction and each thought has an effect. As such, everything that occurs can be explained by the mind as *karma*. A person's *karma* consists of whatever he is presently experiencing, or has yet to experience. These experiences are the results of actions that he has performed, or is now performing, as well as thoughts he has had and now has. When a person is successful in a particular endeavor, or when a pleasant experience befalls him, you may hear it said that "he has good *karma*." The superficial interpretation is "as you sow, so shall you reap." But there is a more profound meaning of "good *karma*." In the classical sense, good *karma* manifests as a force that guides the seeker into those auspicious situations which expose him to and instruct him in the doctrine of Self-Realization. For example, in India, a person born into a spiritual family is said to have exceptionally good *karma*. Similarly, the superficial interpre-

tation of "bad *karma*" is that a person who has accumulated debits for his past thoughts and actions will experience adversities in his worldly life. But the more significant meaning is that a person with negative *karma* will have his realization of Self seriously impeded. He will find it exceedingly difficult to overcome his ignorance and make progress in shaking off the bonds that tie him to the ego. Therefore, in the classical sense, a person may appear highly successful in the world, but may actually be experiencing bad *karma*. If his success, wealth, or lofty position does not result in his "awakening," it is of small value. Conversely, a person whose wordly life is difficult, who might be characterized as having bad *karma* may, exactly because of these difficulties, be led to search for the *cause* of his adversities. This search, causing him to turn inward, can result in his awakening.

Karma, the doctrine of cause and effect, is advanced to also explain reincarnation. Since each action (cause) must, in some way and at some time, manifest as an effect, what will happen if actions are performed and the physical body does not live long enough to experience the result of these actions? What becomes of the multitude of desires that have engendered these actions and that remain ungratified? These do not cease to exist, in the sense that they have no further consequences, just because the physical body is transformed into dust or ashes. The ungratified desires and the result of actions yet to manifest remain in the ego. *It is the ego that reincarnates.* The ego manufactures a new body in which desires and actions can continue their endless cycles. This is why you are not consciously aware of where your desires come from or why you are reaping the results—pleasant and unpleasant—of actions that you do not know you have sown. These things do not befall you out of blind chance. There are no accidents. Everything connected with the ego's projection of the world is cause and effect. The conclusion is this: If desires and the actions they engender are infinite, the physical bodies in which the ego incarnates are also endless. (Words such as "infinite" and "endless" are used in the context of time as an aspect of the ego-world. Self, your true nature, does not exist in the ego's projection of time.) So the ego, with which you have identified and think of as "I," travels perpetually around the circle, experiencing over and over the

manifold conditions of its own projection.

There are three types of *karma*: 1) that which is carried over from previous incarnations and is discharged during this incarnation; 2) that which is carried over from previous incarnations and is not discharged in this incarnation; and 3) that which is generated in this incarnation and, together with the second type, is carried into future incarnations. How will this infinite cycle of births and deaths be terminated? Only by the recognition of Self, which spells automatic annihilation of the ego.

It is usually out of sheer weariness that the sleeping person awakens. That is, having identified with and experienced the conditions of the ego for "as many lifetimes as there are grains of sand on the desert" without experiencing the permanent happiness and peace he is seeking, there occurs some incident—and it can be anything—that causes a momentary jarring. This jarring awakens him, perhaps for only a moment, but the sleeper finds he cannot return to his sleeping state and the process of actively becoming a seeker, as described above, is initiated.

The ignorant person is fascinated by *karma*, not because he

understands it as the need to devote his full energies to escaping from his bondage, but because he wants to know about his past lives and possible future lives. As if he does not have sufficient suffering in this present incarnation, the ignorant person wants to know the pain of previous and future incarnations. There is no end to the ego's tolerance for misery! All efforts to know or speculate about previous incarnations are strongly discouraged by the *Guru*. He advises, "Find out who you are in this incarnation before you seek to know who you were in other incarnations. Incarnations imply that you have been born and that you will die. See if this is really the case." The sleeping person wants to know about past incarnations and about thoughts and actions that constitute "good" and "bad" *karma*. He is like the man in the burning house who, instead of escaping from the fire, wants to determine how the fire started and what type of fire it is. In the course of his examination, he is consumed by the flames. Yoga literature informs us that, in the context of *karma*, an incarnation is rare and precious and one must use it wisely by making all necessary efforts to achieve Self-Realization.

The sleeping person does not

know the source of his desires and accepts them, for the most part, as the natural course of events. From time to time he may question the *types* of desires he is entertaining and may evaluate them as positive or negative, but will never question *the nature of desire itself*. Where do desires come from? Why are they regarded as natural? In truth, desire is not natural; it is a disease. The stronger the desires, the more serious the illness. Desire begets desire without end, and the fever does not abate. A person infected with desire cannot know peace. The awakened person begins to understand how desires confine him permanently in the prison of his ego-mind, and that attempting to terminate desires by gratifying them is like trying to put out a fire with gasoline. When you perceive a desire arising—and it is entirely possible to cultivate such perception—become quiet for a few moments and attempt to feel what is transpiring within. You will recognize a definite disturbance. The stronger the desire, the more intense the disturbance. And these disturbances, in varying degrees of intensity, are incessantly occurring within you like the waves rising from the ocean. Society applauds those who are "highly motivated." But the per-

son with such motivation is driven mercilessly in the world by his ego-mind to gratify his desires. He may, indeed, be able to gratify certain desires, but in the course of his efforts to do so, myriad *new* desires (as is the case with problems) are generated. He is imprisoned in a terrible hell that perpetuates itself. No person who identifies with the ego is ever able to say, "There, that's it. I've satisfied my last desire. Now I'm finished with them and I can relax in peace." The irony, of course, is that a person becomes involved in this relentless process so that he can know happiness and security, but the nature of desire is to spawn additional desire so that there can be no security.

How, then, shall we deal with desires? Do we supress them? No. Desires that are deliberately held in abeyance will bide their time and then manifest with increased ferocity. The procedure is to become aware of desires as they arise and attempt to see *where they are coming from*. Shine your light upon them and try to find their source. Desires are exposed and dissolved by this type of investigation. They will arise with less frequency and less intensity. So, ask them to show you where they come from and by what right

they seize you and make you do their bidding. They will run away, for they have no authority other than that granted to them by the ego, of which they are an aspect. They arise together with the ego. Find that place of origin.

You may think that this investigation will somehow impair your ability to act in the world, to achieve goals, to enjoy life. Such is not the case. Nothing that you need to do in the world will ever be negatively affected by these procedures. At first, this is difficult to understand, because the ego continues its efforts to convince you that it is running the show, that without its desires, thoughts, instructions, and guidance you will become a vegetable, a blithering idiot unable to cope with the necessities. But all necessary action on your part will continue without the ego, because the ego is an interloper, an imposter. A concrete statue of Hercules may show him to be supporting the world on his back. But it is the concrete, not the image of the man, who is the real support. Your Reality, your support, is the concrete; the ego has etched its image in that support. One *Guru* has described the situation this way: If, when riding on a train, you elect to keep your suitcase on your lap rather than place it in the luggage compartment, that is *your* foolishness. The train carries the same weight regardless of where you place your luggage. Likewise, if you elect to believe the fabrication of the ego—that it is responsible for running the show —then you must assume its burden. You carry your luggage on your lap and experience discomfort accordingly. But, in Reality, Self carries all of the weight and in Knowing this you can relinquish the burden of the ego by surrendering it to Self. If desires continue to plague you, attempt to channel these desires into *one* desire: Self-Realization. Hold this desire above all others and they will subside. Ultimately, this one remaining desire is consumed in Self.

4

THE ILLUSION OF "IDENTITY"

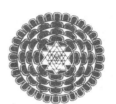

Time-space is also a concept of the mind and arises simultaneously with the projection of the universe. Events occur in time-space; they have a location (space) and a time sequence. The element of time is a necessity for the mind to navigate in the universe. Movement is measured by time and time is measured by movement. Identifying with the mind, it appears that we also experience our existence in a variety of places and in a sequence of time that we perceive as past-present-future. But the Reality of our existence is not in time. A transient, continually changing ego can appear to move in time, but how can eternal, unchanging Self exist in a time dimension? Our Reality is only Now. You can think about the past, but you can do that thinking only Now. Do you ever remember a time in which your Awareness was other than it is Now? You can also think about a future, but you can only do such thinking Now. The future never comes, it is only a thought. You have never had an experience in the future. If the time sequence was Real, you would, each moment, be swept into the past along with the passing moment. But you remain Here and Now. Here and Now is not to be mistaken for the "present" as it is conceived in the past-present-future sequence. There is no such sequence to support your Reality. How can you exist in the present when the present has just now lapsed into the past? A river can serve as an illustration of this. The waters of the river flow, but the river remains the river. Time may flow with the ego, but your Reality is always Now. You move, think, grow, and die in time, but Self engages in none of these dreams.

The mind also functions like a tape recorder. Each thought, event, and action is instantly recorded as it occurs. These millions upon millions of bits of information are stored in the mind-computer's memory. Many can be recalled as required and although this recall can only take place Now, it lends validity to the idea of a past because it appears that you are thinking about actual past events. It is memory that sustains your identification with the ego as a separate, individual self. From its memory banks, the ego will instantly furnish a multitude of facts and statistics about the "you" it has fabricated. Just as you carry various cards and papers to prove that you are who you say you are, memory stores and furnishes information that reinforces the idea that you are a self. But just as the identification card in your wallet is not you but written information *about* you, so is the information furnished by the memory not you. If you investigate the situation, you will conclude that you are always pure Awareness and that you become "you," an individual self with an identity and history only when your memory reminds you of that identity. Because memory is constantly re-establishing and reminding you of your identity, you have accepted it and have mistaken it for your true identity, that of Self. Anxieties about the future are precipitated by memories of past pains and pleasures. Ego feeds you with an abundant supply of these memories so that you are effectively kept off-balance. While you are fluctuating between the nonexistent past and the mirage of the future you cannot be Here, Now.

The illusions of time and memory are emphasized by the Guru in his instruction of the student because the student envisions his Realization as occurring at some future point in time. The Guru informs the student that he cannot expect this to happen, that what he is projecting into a future has already happened and exists Now. Things of the world come and go in time, but Self does not come and go, is not subject to change, and so cannot exist in time. It always IS. Through reiteration of this fact, the Guru literally pushes the student beyond time. Once you have the experience of the timeless state you can never again regard it as Real. Does this affect the way in which you function in the world? Of course not. It is simply that you recognize you never exist in time regardless of what your mind dreams in a past-present-future. You understand your eternal, timeless nature, that you are not subject to birth and death and that Self-Realization always exists Here and Now. Only the ego's super-impositions, with which you have become identified, prevent the Truth from being clearly perceived.

The ego, not satisfied with one identity for you to contend with, manfactures as many as necessary to bind you in its web. For example, it would have you believe that there is a "good" you and a "bad" you, and that it is necessary for the good you to fix up the bad you so that it will become as good as the good you! You say, "I know that I need to improve myself." What has the mind manufactured with that thought? Well, there is an intelligent, good "I" who is standing apart from an inferior "I" and observing that the inferior "I" needs to be improved. Who will do the improving? The intelligent "I" is the observer, detecting the problem but not doing the improving. The inferior "I" is the one who needs improvement; it cannot undertake its own improvement. Therefore, we need an intermediary, a third "I" to act as the improver. And who will judge the progress of the inferior "I"? That is, who will decide if and when the inferior "I" has achieved a satisfactory degree of improvement? We may very well have to call in a fourth "I" for this. And who will judge whether the fourth "I" is correct in its judgement as to whether the inferior "I" has been sufficiently improved? And so on. Not only does the ego maintain a subject-object relationship between you and everything that you perceive as external to you, but it invades your own house and splits it into as many parts as it pleases. In this way it forces you to contend not only with people and conditions of the world, but to fight an internal battle with yourself, as varying degrees of positive I's are pitted against varying degrees of negative I's.

If you observe the way in which you are functioning, you will find that you are always talking to yourself, making plans and telling yourself what to do, as if you were speaking with one or more people. You carry on dialogues among these people. You may have dozens of these characters in your play, each debating with the others regarding the course that will lead to gratification. Each time it is discovered that one of them has failed to navigate properly, he is unseated and another one jumps in for a shot at the wheel. Which of these multiple I's is the real You? The clever one, the deceitful one, the optimist, the religious one, the ambitious one, the angry one, the kind one? None of them. They are all images caused by the ego that appear in the same way you see multiple reflections of yourself when you visit the Hall of Mirrors in the amusement park. The ego divides Self into numerous reflections. When seeing your reflections in these mirrors, you may say, "Look at how I appear in that one, and in that one, and over there!" Which of these images is actually You? None of them. Each one is only a reflection. In a similar way, the ego breaks your Reality into many parts and casts their reflections. You perceive these reflections and identify with them, now with one reflection, now with another. But unlike what transpires in the Hall of Mirrors, you accept the ego's reflections as Real. You are hypnotized by the ego's divisions and you identify with the reflections.

Think of the ego as the glass inserted between the sun and a piece of white paper. The glass splits the sunlight into the spectrum that appears on the white paper. The sun, seeing the colors on the paper says, "Oh, I'm blue. From now on I will exist as blue. No, wait a moment. Look over there. It seems that I'm really red. I have to exist as red. No, wait a moment, I was wrong. I'm actually yellow...." Can the sun be blue, red, yellow, etc.? No, it can only be as it is, pure light. It's reality remains totally unaffected by its identification with the colors. These colors appear as the result of the way in which the glass bends or distorts the light. When the glass is removed the spectrum disappears, not one color at a time, but totally and instantly, and only the pure unbroken light remains. The analogy will serve to illustrate the point: The ego breaks your Reality, Self, into a universe, individual selves and multiple I's within each self. Forgetting that you are Self, you identify with the reflections; you think and act as if they were Real. But no matter how you think and act in your amnesia, Self is unaffected. When the ego, the distortion, is removed your Reality instantly emerges.

These various illustrations—the screen in the movie theater, the river that flows but remains, the reflections in the mirrors, the waves that can never be separate from the ocean, and the glass that bends the light—are attempts to point a finger in the right direction. None of these illustrations are without flaws. But the message should be clear: To find what you are seeking—what you have never lost—it is necessary to retract the mind and senses from the illusions and direct them *inward*.

Society cherishes the concept of self-improvement and places such positive emphasis upon it that one who fails to actively undertake such improvements is usually made to feel inadequate (the ego relies heavily on guilt). The Yogi informs us that one must do whatever is necessary to perform one's duties and if "improvement" enters into these duties, do what you must do. But understand that there is no end to such improvements, because, in order to protect its position, the ego will never permit you to believe that you are totally improved and nothing further is necessary. As

we have seen, it invents numerous bad I's that the good I's need to reform. The ego may have you think it is allied with you in your "good guy" corner, ready to assist you in taking care of the "bad guys." But that is one of its deceits. It secretly has as much affection for the bad guys as it does for the good guys because they're all its offspring, and as quickly as you overcome one bad I, another springs up to take its place.

People will say that they are attempting to overcome a "bad habit." From Yoga philosophy we learn that all habits, personality traits, and behavioral patterns that are regarded both as favorable and unfavorable, constructive and destructive, proceed from one source. For the Yoga student, there is no advantage in examining and attempting to eliminate one bad habit at a time because, as we have noted, there is no end to bad habits. You will never finish with them. Remember that the entity that is examining the habits and evaluating them is the same entity that is manufacturing them! Examining your habits, personality, and behavior is like a magician examining an illusion he has created. Your illusion of existing as an individual self is reinforced through self-analysis. Do you need to examine each

piece of garbage before you dispose of it? Throw out the garbage, the self, and be done with it all at once. When the projector in the theater is turned off, all of the good and bad action that has been occurring on the screen, and all the actors who are portraying good and bad roles disappear instantaneously. The bad ones don't disappear first, or disappear one by one, or disappear a little bit at a time. When the medium through which the illusion is manifesting (the projector) is turned off, the entire illusion is gone all at once. Find your projector, find the source of the ego and put an end to *all* your illusions with one stroke.

5
ACTION WITHOUT KARMA

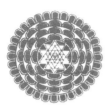

The ego wants and needs regular approval. Being an imposter, it is always insecure and anxious about its position. So it reinforces its pretended reality by having other egos tell it that it is real, through various types of recognition, including commending it on its qualities, whatever they may be. It loves compliments on its nice physical appearance and will frequently go to absurd lengths to receive them. Many egos spend the greater part of an incarnation seeking to have their bodies admired. The ego's desperate need for approval forces you into numerous relationships and situations that have no value for Realization; indeed, they usually are diversionary, consuming much time and energy. With a little thought, many of these will be obvious. Society exhorts you to "get involved," but the *Guru* advises the seeker to be very cautious about involvements. Society wants you to improve yourself, become a better person, go back to school, volunteer your services, attend meetings, make new friends, learn to communicate, and become involved in a myriad of other activities. But the *Guru* cautions: Be acutely aware of what role the ego plays in these things. Do not do anything for approval. Approval only reinforces the pre-

tension of the ego. And offer your own approval to others only as an expression of genuine appreciation, not because the ego is seeking something in return. The discriminating seeker knows when something comes to him that must be done. He does it to the best of his ability, but never *looks* for things to do. When it is possible to do so, the seeker associates with those who, like himself understand the doctrine and seek enlightenment. He attempts to avoid those egos and situations that emit negative vibrations and drain his *prana.*

Society takes a dim view of this type of discrimination. It would characterize the life of a seeker as "selfish." The implication is that when you turn inward, in the way we have been discussing in these pages, you are selfish. And when you are involved in an activity such as helping others, you are unselfish. The fact is that if you are not acting from the center of the circle, the ego is in command, reinforcing itself and gaining approval, and you are totally selfish no matter what you are doing. But manifesting Self, you cannot be selfish regardless of what you are doing, because it is not the ego who performs the actions. The actions flow through you without being distorted by

the ego. This type of pure, selfless action bears no consequences; *because it is free of cause and effect, it generates no karma!* When you perform actions not to achieve results, there is no cause and effect. When the ego's law of cause and effect is overturned, *karma* is terminated. You act, you do what you must do, but there is no sense of *I am helping, I am teaching, I am being kind.* If there is no *I*, no ego in your actions, there can be no consequences, because there is nothing upon which consequences can impact. This subtle and profound doctrine —inaction in action—is the basis for what is designated as *Karma Yoga* and is the essence of India's great scripture, the *Bhagavad Gita.* The principle of action without karma is worthy of your most serious consideration.

Approval and improvement frequently are the incentives for one to sally forth into the world to improve it, to make it a better place in which to live. That is, the ego, seeing the world as imperfect, appoints itself as the agent to help perfect it. (There are certain egos who don't just want to help but have decided to take on the entire job themselves.) The reality of imperfection is reinforced on a second-to-second basis by the media and almost all with whom you come in contact. You are informed, loud and clear, that the world is in terrible condition, disaster is imminent, and madmen are running amok everywhere. But all is not necessarily lost. You are also made to know that although man has wreaked havoc, he can extricate himself from the chaos. This dictim effectively keeps you in a state of acute anxiety which allows the ego to remind you that man's ingenuity (itself) must take charge of the situation if the world is to be saved. So, the ego fabricates chaos and then convinces you that it will cope with the chaos. Existing in a state of insecurity, anxiety, and confusion, not knowing Who or Where he is, a man is nonetheless given to believe that he has the capacity and responsibility to fix up the world. Is the world imperfect, or is your vision imperfect? You will discover, possibly to your astonishment, that as your inner vision is clarified, the world magically improves. Indeed, it improves to the exact extent that you recognize Who you Are! If you want to see your reflection in the mirror place its hand on its head, you must place your hand on your head. If you want to see perfection in the world, you must see your own perfection.

6

THE FALSE GOD OF THE EGO

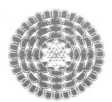

"Self" is another word for "God." This is the God who is the Absolute, immutable, without qualities, pure Awareness, without beginning or end. Self, God, is your Reality. "You Are That." Self is not the God that the ego conceives. The ego, which limits and distorts, invents a God that must also be limited and distorted, as it is a reflection of its inventor. The ego imputes to Self the qualities of its own God and convinces you that God is an entity with emotions (kind, compassionate, but also angry and vengeful), with hopes and ambitions, subject to being pleased and disappointed, with plans that may succeed or fail. The ego concept of God's "purpose and plan" for His creation has been prevalent throughout the ages. Because the ego-mind conceives and attempts to implement "plans" for self-gratification, this planning activity becomes anthropomorphic and is superimposed upon Self, God. God is conceived in the image of the ego: Man, in his ego state, has plans with purposes, so, of course, God must have plans with purposes. But a plan is subject to success and failure, and God is not of the nature of success and failure. He does not work out a plan to unfold in a space-time continuum. No plan was conceived and implemented by Him at some point in the past, no plan is now working out in the present and no plan will be concluded at some point in an illusionary future. All always IS, Here and Now. The mind produces cause and effect and transforms one thing into another. Self, your true nature, does not transform.

The ego may also fabricate one or more "purposes" for your life. Because of the way the mind plays with the elements of the world—influencing and affecting one another—it concludes that these relationships must be purposeful, that something must result from their interaction and that something else must result from that result and so on forever. It also implies that someday, when enough facts have been uncovered, we will at last know the "purpose" of life. Of course, no such time will ever arrive, because purpose and time are inventions of the mind. There will always be more facts to uncover, more discoveries to be made. So you may come to believe that, even though you can't put your finger on it, there must be some purpose for your existence.

The mind is greatly disturbed when we challenge its cherished concept of "purpose." "If there's no purpose," it whines, "then what's it all for anyhow?" The

Truth is that it's not *for* anything. Existence, Awareness IS. You ARE. Is that not purpose enough? Could there be any more significant purpose? It is the mind that asks, "Why was I born? What is the purpose of my life? Why was the world created? What is God's plan for the world and for mankind?" As Self, you understand that these questions are meaningless; they disappear the moment one awakens. When you dream during sleep, you are totally immersed in the creations of your dream. They involve you in many situations and you have many experiences. But when you awaken, you don't question what happened to the people in your dream. Usually, you forget them immediately, but even if they are remembered they have no further meaning for you. In the same way the questions about existence that hold such great concern in the ego state vanish in Self-Realization.

Does this mean that we do not do what we can to relieve suffering and misery? Again, of course not. We do, to the best of our ability, whatever comes to us to do, but our compassion and love are expressed in *selfless action*. We act without anticipating results, without seeking approval, without feeling we are an instrument carrying out some purpose

in an incomprehensible plan. If we do not, as yet, have a complete recognition of Self, we perform our actions to the best of our understanding—derived from study and meditation—of the Self-Realized state.

The sleeping person believes the self to be real. Therefore, the protection and inflation of this self (ego) becomes the business of his life. He seeks pleasure without pain, growth without decay, happiness without sorrow, success without failure. Because the sleeper fails to understand the nature of the ego, he believes that these things are possible, that he can grab hold of one end of the stick and remove it from the opposite end. But there are always two ends to the stick, no matter how long or short it may be. Similarly, in the ego's projection of duality, pain is inherent in pleasure, sorrow in happiness, and failure in success. One cannot be known without, sooner or later, the other being experienced. These opposites are continually transformed from one to the other in varying degrees. You judge your degree of success by the failure you have experienced or that you imagine could be experienced. You evaluate your present happiness by the degree of past sorrows (as furnished by the computer's memory). But the sleeping person, even while becoming aware of these alternating opposites, continues to strive for what he perceives as the "positive" aspect of life and fights desperately to avoid what will threaten or diminish the ego, perceived as the "negative" aspect. These efforts, which cannot possibly succeed, are frequently cloaked in the respectable guise of "providing for my family," or "getting ahead in life." The ego, masquerading in these noble disguises, prevents the sleeping person from understanding that taking care of his family has nothing to do with the way in which the ego is manuevering him and that *he will always be exactly where he must be and always have exactly what he needs.* The awakened person is usually able to recognize this Truth relatively early in the meditation practice and this awareness relieves him of a tremendous burden. The ego superimposes itself upon all that transpires and will interject its concepts of "free will" as opposed to "destiny." These again are two ends of the same stick. Self, your Reality, has nothing to do with what the ego interprets as "free will" and "destiny." Remove the ego and you have pure action without cause and effect.

Does the Self-Realized person have preferences and make choices? Because he *appears* to act in the same way as all people, it is concluded that his actions also are based on choices. But, being devoid of ego, *everything flows through him.* There is no "I" to evaluate an action as a choice that has been made among many possibilities. He is in a state of *choiceless awareness.* What IS, IS. "I AM THAT I AM." The splitting of this One, Whole, ISness into the illusion of possibilities and making you believe that what you observe or experience is the result of your having made a choice among many possibilities, is the work of the ego. Just as it divides the sun into the spectrum, the ego divides what IS into a multiple of possibilities and choices. It reinforces its reality of these possibilities by frequently informing you that you have made the *wrong* choice. Even so, the sleeping person seldom questions the mind's ability to eventually put everything right. The ego-mind nominates itself as the entity that will provide all necessary guidance. It seconds its own nomination and elects itself unanimously.

Frequently, the sleeping person is lured by the promise of psychic powers and ESP (extrasensory perception). These things deserve some attention here. Because so-called "extrasensory perception" is an aspect of the ego's subtle planes and the ordinary person is consciously functioning on the gross plane, where he is involved primarily with the physical universe, the subtle plane is not consciously known to him. Therefore, he speaks of this unfamiliar level of perception as "extra." When the gross, outward-flowing senses that cognize the external world are turned inward, they become subtle. Clairvoyance, for example, is external sight turned inward. None of these subtle perceptions are really "extra." They are wholly contained within the universe of the microcosm that is the subtle body of each person. To most, however, they remain consciously unknown. During the course of Yoga and related practices, these subtle planes are contacted. But it is only the ill-advised person who will involve himself with these planes for purposes of gratification. In the strongest possible terms, the Guru cautions the student against involvement with visions and powers, since they can have the most adverse effect on the student's development. The ignorant person is highly desirous of uncovering, cultivating, and utilizing such powers, because through them he envisions himself controlling, influencing, and manipulating people and conditions. He desires all this exactly because he *is* ignorant. He has no comprehension that such powers are utterly useless and actually are obstacles to attaining Self-Realization. He is consciously unaware of seeking Self (although that is all that each person does). If the doctrine of Self is explained to him, the ignorant person has not yet "ears to hear." He remains asleep, dreaming of power, control, and manipulation to gratify his senses and ego in an illusionary world. To him, such power may lie in ESP. So, although asleep to his real nature, he attempts to cultivate "powers" so that he may enhance his life.

The seeker, the awakened person, understands the nature of the quest. He recognizes that Self manifests when he discards, eliminates, and transcends all that is of the not-Self. If he consciously seeks to accomplish anything, it is not to acquire but to *discard*. Any need to cultivate ESP, that is, to use the projections of the ego in a more subtle way, is totally absent. All desire to influence people and events, on whatever plane, no matter how noble the motives or objective, binds you to the not-Self, thereby petuating your suffering. So the *Guru* advises to observe with *detachment* any such phenomena that may manifest during the course of practice. They can be regarded as signposts along the way that indicate the inward journey is proceeding, that the mind and senses have been sufficiently refined to make contact with the subtle planes. Like a traveler who stops at a tavern, becomes intoxicated, and is unable to continue to his destination all preoccupation with subtle phenomena will abort your journey and is to be absolutely avoided.

7

FUNCTION OF THE GURU

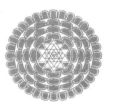

The Yoga practice requires no deliberate changes in your work or relationships. All continues as it has. The modifications produced by Yoga are internal and practically imperceptible to another person. The process is a metamorphosis, similar to the way a caterpillar is transformed into a butterfly. The work that is going on within is very personal; it is extremely difficult to speak of it and the true seeker will be most reluctant to discuss what is occurring. Realization seems to develop in silence with minimal disturbance. Periods of silent meditation, as presented in the Meditation section, are essential. When a diver seeks a treasure at the bottom of the sea, he is unable to speak. Upon returning to the surface with the treasure, he joyfully describes his good fortune and is able to tell others where the treasure was found. While the seeker searches for Self he is disinclined to discuss his quest, but once having attained Realization is able to instruct others from his own experience.

Realization does not preclude the *memory* of illusion. The enlightened person knows, and is better able than anyone, to point out the nature of the illusion. A recovered drug addict does not need to be experiencing hallucina-

tions to help an addict who is having these delusions. The memory of the hallucinating experience remains for the one who has recovered, but the delusion has no power to cause suffering. Similarly, the Self-Realized person performs his duties and meets all of his responsibilities and obligations, but the way he regards these things is totally different from the sleeping (hallucinating) person. He does not perform actions to achieve anything, because he has nothing further to achieve. Success and failure, gain and loss, have no effect on him because he has transcended these continually alternating opposites. He knows unconditioned joy because his existence is spontaneous and new each moment and not dependent upon memory. He may laugh and cry along with others, but his pleasure and sorrow move from Self's love and compassion, not from ego. Others see this person as a separate, individual being, but he sees none apart from himself.

Perhaps the most compelling quality of the enlightened person is a sense of peace—equanimity and balance—that is felt in his presence. He transmits calm, unperturbed vibrations to those around him, and the student can understand what the ancients taught: "Neither rejoice in your good fortune nor despair in your travail." They were advising the seeker to maintain quiescence, to minimize life's "ups" and "downs" by regarding what befalls him with dispassion, knowing that everything furthers his or her development. You may interpret this dispassionate view as detracting from the joy or fun of living. But even what your mind envisions as the wildest joy is short-lived and is soon transformed into sorrow. The greatest happiness that one derives from conditions of the world is but the palest reflection of the sublime Bliss of Self. Understand that when you seek happiness in the conditions of the world, you are really seeking reintegration with your true state of Unconditioned Bliss. Joy is the property only of Self. There is no joy in the ego. Whatever happiness you experience in the world is the Happiness of Self *filtered through the ego.* Cultivating equilibrium, balance, in your everyday activities leads to the experience of Self and is, therefore, strongly advocated by the *Guru.*

The Self-Realized person may not make his Realization known in an overt way. Or he may actively engage in instruction, in which case he is referred to as a *Guru.* Literally translated, a *Guru* is "one who dispells darkness." (The words "darkness" and "ignorance" are not used derogatorily, but rather to describe the state of the sleeping person.) Yoga literature leaves no doubt that the true *Guru* is *within* and it is He who awakens you. But because the beginning student still identifies with his body and is unable to hear the inner instruction, he looks for a *Guru* who also has a body; he seeks the *Guru* externally. "When the student is ready, the master will appear" is an axiom of Yoga. This axiom is communicated to the student so that he will continue to prepare through study and practice, and not become obsessed with an active external search for the *Guru.*

Gurus present their teachings in many situations. Some are wanderers (as were Jesus and Buddha) and teach where and how they will. Some arrange a schedule of appearances at one or more places. Some have one or more *ashrams* (retreats) and travel among them. Some remain permanently at one *ashram.* Also, there are *Gurus* who remain isolated and guide without being physically present in the student's environment. All this is a matter of the style of the particular *Guru.*

The function of the *Guru* is to push the student within so that the internal *Guru* may pull him to Self. Each external *Guru* utilizes his own techniques to effect this "push." Such techniques include personal contact, lectures, discussions, rituals, *mantrams,* initiations, and meditations. The student may take as much time as he wishes in selecting his *Guru.* That is, the student may encounter a number of Self-Realized teachers none of whom have the necessary strong attraction. But if and when he *is* attracted, drawn toward the *Guru* as if by a magnet, and is accepted as a disciple, he must surrender himself to the *Guru* and trust him implicitly. The student must follow the *Guru's* instructions without question. He may question the *Guru* about all things of the world, but not about his instructions. The *Guru,* exactly because he *is* a *Guru,* knows what is necessary for the student's enlightenment and issues his instructions accordingly. The *Guru* has no wish to enter into a protracted teacher-student relationship. Although his commitment to the disciple is as total as is the disciple's commitment to him, and he assumes certain responsibilities for the disciple's development, the *Guru* wants the disciple to become his own teacher as quickly as possible. But this depends on the level of the disciple's understanding of the guidance he receives. The disciple may maintain the relationship for as long as is necessary. The *Guru* never portrays himself as being indispensable; rather constantly conveys to the disciple that he is only a reflection of the disciple's inner *Guru* and encourages him to contact that *Guru*. More and more the disciple is pushed into seeking inner guidance. When Self is attained, the disciple realizes that all along he and the *Guru* have been One.

How does one encounter a *Guru* in the Western world? The situation is no different than in the East. When the student is ready, the teacher will appear. How will you know that this person is truly enlightened, that he or she can provide the necessary instruction? Trust your inner guidance, it always Knows. If you begin a relationship with one teacher and find that he or she has given you all that he or she may have to offer *you*, can you change to another teacher? Absolutely. A true teacher will always encourage this and may, if he or she sees it necessary, suggest it. Learn to listen for and trust your inner guidance. It is always there and will respond when you make contact. Turn inward, become very quiet

and listen. The voice is always guiding you; be patient until it comes through clearly. How do you know that the guidance is genuine and not a trick of the mind, a type of self-hypnosis? It is unmistakably genuine. It is more Real than any instruction or guidance you have ever received in the external world.

Can you undertake such a relationship with a teacher and/or pursue your Yoga practice amidst what frequently appear to be overwhelming distractions in your everyday life? Yes, you can and you must. As previously stated, an incarnation is rare and precious. It is only on this plane that Self-Realization can be achieved. The other planes, those experienced during that state we call "death," are for the discharge of *karma*, pleasant and unpleasant. The mind cannot be consciously altered on these planes; the necessary practice cannot be pursued.

The awakened person soon learns how to implement his practice in the world. Certain suggestions for this are offered in the Meditation section. You attempt to remain awake and refuse to be hypnotized by activity. You remember to discriminate between the Real and the not-Real, the Self and the not-Self. You are not deceived by appearances, but look

for the *source* of the appearance. One is inclined to see the *forms* of objects made from clay, while losing sight of the clay itself. The senses are hypnotized by the forms, but the forms cannot exist without the clay. When the forms are altered, or the objects destroyed, the clay remains. In the same way, when the world and all that appears to exist in it (forms) are seen by the ego, they are an illusion. But seen as Self (clay), All is Real.

8

YOGA, THE UNIVERSAL PRACTICE FOR HERE AND NOW

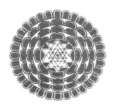

There are many paths on which people travel to God-Consciousness, Self-Realization. Yoga is one such path. Within itself, Yoga encompasses various paths and techniques and each has its own *Gurus*. Yoga is the mergence of what, at this moment, you regard as "I" with that which is your Reality, which we have designated "Self." The word "Yoga" is used to describe both the means and the end. When it is said that you are practicing Yoga, it means you are using the techniques of Yoga to achieve Yoga (Self-Realization). These techniques include the practice of *Hatha*, observation and control of the breath, selfless action, meditation, self-surrender, tracing the mind to its source, and others. In a sense, everything can be considered as an avenue to Self, but because specific techniques have been successfully taught and applied for many centuries, these are emphasized in the Yoga practice. The techniques are not mutually exclusive. Various ones can be practiced together. For example, on a daily basis you can practice your postures and breathing exercises, and follow this with a period of meditation. During your daily activities, experiment with the selfless action that has been described, and when you find

yourself in any quiet situation during the day, retract your mind and attempt to follow it inward to the place from which it arises. (This technique is described in the Meditation section.) The objective is to remind yourself as often as possible of the practice, because it can be so easily pushed into the background when you are immersed in your worldly activities. If you are not alert, you will find that significant periods of time can elapse without your paying attention to what we have described as the real business of life.

There need be no conflict between Yoga and one's religion. All religions proclaim the omniscience of God, Self, and most teach the importance of ego-annihilation. Moses, David, Solomon, the prophets, Jesus—these were the *Gurus* of the Old and New Testaments. They incarnated as guides to Self. They instructed those who were awakening, who had "eyes to see and ears to hear." Moses, Buddha, Jesus, Mohammed, Ramakrishna and many others taught the doctrine of Self-Realization to diverse groups at different times and in widely varying circumstances. Because the teachings were directed to the level of understanding among the people of diverse civilizations,

there may appear to be differences in what was taught. But these differences are superficial. All *Gurus* speak as Self. If you examine their teachings from this perspective, there can be no contradiction or conflict. Self is devoid of differentiation. The superficial distinctions in the teachings have been accentuated through misinterpretations by those who came afterward and who did not possess the pure Knowledge of Self. The distinctions became the basis for all manner of doctrinal structures around which multitudes of peoples were organized. In the name of "truth," declaring that *its* distinction is more genuine than the other distinctions, the adherents of one group have slaughtered those of others. The ego encourages this insanity. But the teachings of the *Guru*, Messiah, Prophet, and Enlightened One are not affected by how their "followers" have interpreted them. The teachings remain as absolute Truth, as a guide to and description of the state of Self-Realization. To understand your religion, absorb the *original words* of He upon whom it was founded.

Hatha Yoga cannot be in conflict with any religion. Nor can observation of the breath, quieting the mind, selfless action, fixing the attention on a given object. No deity, worship, ritual ceremony, or prayer is involved in the practices presented in this book. Of whom are the thousands of Yoga classes in the Western world composed? There are very few Hindus. These classes are attended by Protestants, Catholics, Jews, and the adherents of just about any other religion and sect we might name. Yoga presents the doctrine of Self; it seeks no converts.

The strong attraction that Yoga currently holds for so many people is that it not only describes the process and state of Self-Realization in very *direct* terms, but its practices are so diverse that they can appeal to all natures. Those who are inclined toward the physical, intellectual, mystical, or emotional can engage in techniques of that Yoga, or those Yogas, that seem most pertinent. These techniques are not fads or recent innovations. They have been applied with great success for thousands of years by millions of people, and the practitioner can experience what it is they purport to accomplish in a relatively brief period of serious application.

Regular readings of this Philosophy section will assist you in an intellectual understanding of the subject and will act as the "push"

that we have mentioned in connection with the work of the *Guru*. The more you reflect on these matters, the more the mind is turned inward and illumined by the light of Self.

MEDITATION

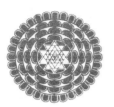

An intellectual understanding of Yoga philosophy is extremely helpful, but cannot, by itself, result in the enlightenment we are seeking. To dissolve the ego, meditation is essential.

There is nothing mysterious or difficult about Yoga meditation. It is not involved with self-hypnosis, extrasensory perception, occult powers, or a "trip." It is not introspection in the sense of self-analysis. It is not prayer. It is the simple act of sitting quietly for a comfortable interval and directing the mind and senses in a way that will enable you to confirm for yourself the Truth of what has been indicated in the previous pages: Your Reality, your true nature, is other than what you have believed it to be. In the course of understanding what you are not, what you Are emerges.

Our initial objective in the meditation practice is to control the wildness of the mind. If we can begin to quiet the mind and reduce the frequency of thoughts, there is the possibility of seeing beyond the mind. When a pool of water is disturbed by vibrations, you cannot see beyond the surface. But once these vibrations have ceased, our view of the bottom is clear. In the same way, the vibrations caused by incessant thoughts obscure the view of Reality that is our essence. To gain the inner vision of this Reality, the mind must be quieted. But the mind is like a wild horse that has run free for its entire life and will fiercely resist all attempts to be restrained. The restraint must be gentle, methodical, and persistent. In our Yoga meditation, this restraint is accomplished by supplying the mind with a focal point. The wild horse may be slowly enticed into the corral with food, and gradually will submit to those who wish to tame him. Similarly, the mind can be lured into quietude by meditation that it finds interesting, that it does not perceive as a threat and want to run away from; gradually it will submit to control. When this control is achieved, the thoughts subside and the place from where thoughts arise can be recognized. It is at this point that the individual self, the ego, merges with Reality and Yoga is accomplished.

In the following pages a variety of classical meditation techniques are presented. It is suggested that you experiment with each to determine which is most effective for achieving the quieting objective. Minds and personalities are different (individual inclination and tendencies are attributed to *karma*, the thoughts and actions of innumerable previous incarnations), and they will react differently to the various techniques. That technique that holds the most attraction, that proves to be both interesting and easy to work with, will be the most effective and is the one you should utilize. Here is the suggested procedure: Immediately following your *Hatha* Yoga routine of the day, practice *Observation of the Breath* and then work with the first meditation technique. On the next day, following your *Hatha* practice, work with the second technique and so forth until you have gone through all. (Keep a schedule of the technique to be practiced on each day.) Then return to the first technique and work through the entire group a second and third time. As you go along, make a note of which techniques are interesting to you and seem to have an effect. After you have gone through the group for the third time, select two or three that have proven of value. Then, work with that selected group—one each day—until one emerges as your principal technique. From that point on, utilize only the chosen technique. As occurs with the *Hatha asanas*, there will be days on which you do well and days on which you seem to have setbacks. This is the natural process. Make no attempt to evaluate your progress in meditation; simply practice your technique as you would any exercise. At some point the breakthrough will occur and it will be unmistakable. No description of this experience is possible. Patience and regularity are indispensable. You must attempt to practice each day, whether or not you feel like practicing.

Although the horse is enticed by the food, he is still cautious. If the mind suspects a serious attempt is being made to restrain and control it, it will attempt to flee. This takes the form of it diverting you with a multitude of excuses as to why you should not engage in the meditation practice: You don't have time, you have something else to do that's more important, you'll do it later, you're not making progress, you're tired etc. This is all nonsense. The mind senses a threat to its position of total dominance and it has no wish to preside over its own dissolution. But remember that each time you practice meditation you shine a light on the shadow of the ego. A shadow cannot withstand light, and as the intensity of your light increases through meditation practice, the ego's reality fades accordingly.

In certain techniques, objects are required. Be sure to have the pertinent object on hand before beginning your *Hatha* practice because meditation should immediately follow the *asanas*.

OBSERVATION OF THE BREATH

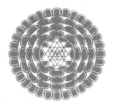

In all but one of the following meditation practices, it is suggested that you observe your breathing for two minutes.

Sit in a Lotus posture and simply direct your full attention to the manner in which you are breathing. As you note the rhythm of your breathing, it gradually will become slower. When the tempo decreases, the rate of heartbeat, pulse, and other physical functions are correspondingly slowed. Because the mind has a direct connection with the breath, it too is quieted. This condition of quietude enables you to undertake serious meditation. If you become aware that your mind is wandering, return it to the breathing.

When approximately two minutes have elapsed, go on to the meditation practice.

YANTRA

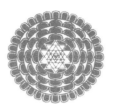

A *yantra* is a geometric symbol with special properties. It imparts energy to the subtle body and is utilized for expanding the consciousness. Also, its symmetry is said to pull together diverse elements of the individual ego and integrate them in a way that facilitates one-pointed concentration. An ancient and highly effective *yantra* that we will utilize is the circle with a dot in the center. Prior to your *Hatha* session, have this *yantra* on hand. On a piece of white paper or white cardboard, preferably 8½"x11" or larger, use dark ink or a marker to draw a circle. You can approximate a circle; it need not be perfect. Next, approximate the center of the circle and place an easily seen small circle there. Fill in the small circle so that it is solid.

1. Place the *yantra* at a distance where it will be easily seen from where you will be seated on your mat.

2. Sit in one of the Lotus postures (23 in the *Hatha* Yoga section).

3. Practice Observation of the Breath for approximately two minutes.

4. Fix your gaze on the *yantra*. Hold it steadily on the *yantra* for approximately two minutes. Both your gaze and attention must remain fully focused on the figure.

If your gaze remains fixed, but the attention wanders, this technique will not be effective. Each time you become aware that other thoughts are intruding, dismiss them and redirect your full attention to the *yantra*. In the beginning you will find other thoughts continually attempting to divert you, so be alert. The only way to achieve one-pointed concentration on the *yantra*, and in all of the meditation techniques, is to patiently dismiss the intruding thoughts. This constant intrusion will indicate to you that although you earnestly wish to focus your full attention on the *yantra*, the extraneous thoughts, like a spoiled child, force themselves upon you and demand your attention. In other words, this totally uncontrolled thought process is occurring throughout your lifetime and unless you practice to achieve control, as described above, your thoughts will maintain their complete domination of your existence.

5. Following the two minute period, close your eyes. Now visualize the identical figure with closed eyes for approximately three additional minutes, or for as long as you wish. If the image begins to fade, make it reappear by mentally drawing the circumference of the circle in a clockwise direction and then place the dot in the center. Any color in which the *yantra* appears is satisfactory. If the visualizations are impossible or extremely weak, reinforce the image by opening your eyes and observing the figure for a brief period. Then close your eyes and make another attempt. By continuing this procedure, you will develop the necessary strength for visualization.

6. Open your eyes, slowly extend your legs and rest a few moments before arising. This *yantra* may be visualized in any situation where you have the opportunity to close your eyes for a few minutes. It quiets the mind and revitalizes the subtle body.

OM

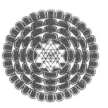

As a *yantra* results in heightened awareness through visual concentration, a *mantra* produces this state through audio vibrations. A *mantra* is a special sequence of Sanskrit letters and syllables, usually of ancient origin, that is intoned in a series of repetitions. And as a *yantra* may be visualized with the eyes closed, a *mantra* may be intoned inwardly, that is, without sound that is externally audible. For this audio meditation, we will use what is acknowledged as the *supreme mantra*: OM. The effect of this powerful *mantra* can be immediately felt.

1. Sit in a Lotus posture. Practice Observation of the Breath for approximately two minutes.

2. Once you understand these directions, keep your eyes closed during the practice. Exhale deeply. Inhale slowly and deeply.

3. Divide your exhalation into halves. During the first half, intone the word "Oh" in a low, steady, audible tone. There must be force and energy in the sound and it must be intoned slowly with control. Your voice should not weaken or waver.

4. When you have reached the halfway point in your breath, close the lips and pronounce the letter "Mmmmmmmmmm" in the same low, steady, controlled, forceful tone. The sound should vibrate throughout your body like the buzzing of a bee. Do not permit the sound to trail off and become weak as you reach the end of your breath.

5. Without pause, inhale slowly and deeply and repeat. Perform seven times.

6. Beginning with the eighth inhalation, perform silent repetitions of OM. Your breathing remains the same, but the mouth is closed and the sound is not produced with the voice but is heard with the inner ear. Attempt to hear the identical sounds that you produced audibly during the first seven repetitions. At all times your consciousness must be totally fixed on the external and internal sounds. Do not permit the repetitions to become automatic while your mind wanders.

7. Following the final repetition, keep your eyes closed for a brief period and become aware of what is transpiring within.

OM may be inaudibly practiced in any situation where you have the opportunity to close your eyes for a few minutes. As your ability grows in concentration, external sounds will not disturb you and you will be able to hear the silent OM whenever you wish. You may eventually discern that the OM sound is continual within you and you do not need to intone it, but only to tune in to it! OM can become a highly effective technique for relief of anxiety and stress.

CANDLE

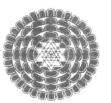

The flame of a candle provides an excellent object for meditation. The eyes are attracted to the flame and the gaze can be easily fixed upon it. It makes a strong impression upon the retina and this is retained for a relatively lengthy period when the eyes are closed. The light generated from the flame when the gaze is fixed on it—and then retained when the eyes are closed—produces a condition of heightened awareness. It is as if the light that is transmitted actually illuminates the consciousness. It is important to note that the element of light appears in numerous descriptions of spirituality, and Self-Realization is frequently characterized in terms of light: illumination, enlightenment, radiance, brilliance. Candle meditation imparts a sense of this illumined state.

1. Place a lighted candle approximately three feet from your mat. Sit in a Lotus posture and practice Observation of the Breath for approximately two minutes.

2. Fix your gaze steadily upon the flame and hold it there for approximately two minutes, blinking as necessary. Continue to dismiss all intruding thoughts and hold your full attention on the flame.

3. Now close your eyes and place your palms over them. Keep the hands and arms relaxed because they must remain in this position for approximately three minutes. Retain the image of the flame. Hold it as steady as possible and do not allow your attention to wander. If the flame begins to fade, use your concentration to bring it back. If it becomes very weak, or fades entirely, open your eyes and gaze at the flame for a brief period. Then close your eyes and resume the practice.

4. When, after several practice sessions, you have become proficient in retaining the image with closed eyes, add this technique: Use your concentration to slowly bring the flame forward. Continue to slowly bring it forward until you *merge* with it, until you are absorbed by it. At this point there is no longer you and a flame; the subject-object condition is terminated; there is only LIGHT. Remain in this state as long as you wish.

5. Open your eyes, extend your legs and rest a few moments before rising.

ALTERNATE NOSTRIL BREATHING

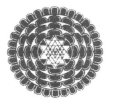

We have learned this technique in the *Hatha* Yoga section (26) as one that serves as a powerful natural tranquilizer. However, for serious Yoga students, Alternate Nostril Breathing is practiced in the context of meditation. (Remember that meditation is not relaxation in the usual sense; it is *acute awareness*.) Simply breathing through the nostrils alternately balances the positive-negative ratio of the *prana* (life-force) as it enters and leaves the body, and induces a state of equilibrium. We have spoken of the need for equilibrium in the Philosophy section. It is frequently the case that in this state of balance, the thoughts will automatically cease to invade the consciousness and the student is able to temporarily experience the quiet joy of the thoughtless state. The importance of this experience is that it acts as an incentive for the student to achieve this condition at will, to be able to turn off the thoughts and rest the mind and senses. While this state is not our ultimate objective, it is a milestone on the path.

For the purpose of meditation, the counting that we previously learned in Alternate Nostril Breathing must be modified. It is a more difficult count and will require practice, but your efforts will be well worthwhile.

1. Observation of the Breath need not be practiced. Refer to 26 in the *Hatha* Yoga section. You are seated in a Lotus posture, and the way you will breathe through the nostrils alternately remains exactly the same as described. However, the count of 8-4-8; 8-4-8 is now changed to 4-16-8; 4-16-8. To accommodate this count, you must inhale more quickly (but as silently as possible), and retain the inhalation longer. The exhalation count of 8 is the same as previously learned. It will require some practice to get this new rhythm flowing smoothly.

2. Perform seven rounds. Keep your eyes closed throughout. Your attention must be fully focused on the counting and the flow of the breath (*prana*) as it enters, is retained, and is expelled. Do not permit the counting and breathing to become automatic while your mind wanders.

3. Following the final round, return your hand to your knee. Keep your eyes closed and become aware of the feeling of perfect equilibrium—almost a floating sensation—you are experiencing. This is the condition that should be maintained during your daily activities.

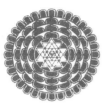

FLOWER

In the Philosophy section it was stated that the mind can never truly Know anything. It can only know *about* things in a perpetual subject-object relationship. It cannot Know because it must remain outside, apart from the object it is examining. In order to Know, one must become that which it seeks to Know; the mind must *merge* with and dissolve in what appears to be external to it. The flower is the object we will use to experiment with such merging. Any flower you obtain for this purpose is satisfactory. As with the candle, the flower is a compelling object upon which to fix the gaze. It is beautiful, colorful, has intricate patterns and textures, and it has the qualities of life: birth, growth, decay. (In the absence of a flower, a small house plant can be substituted.)

1. Place the flower in a vase or other container approximately three feet from your mat. Sit in a Lotus posture. Practice Observation of the Breath for approximately two minutes.

2. During the next ten minutes you are to become involved with the flower to the extent that none of the other senses and thoughts will distract your attention. Visually examine its structure, form, texture, and color. Attempt to discern the smallest detail of each.

Take your time. Your concentration must be total. If you perceive that other thoughts are intruding, dismiss them patiently but firmly. Remember that this process is like disciplining a spoiled child who will eventually respond to your directions if you issue them patiently, firmly, repeatedly. You will be able to merge with the flower to the extent that your concentration remains fixed. That is, if your mind and vision have been totally involved with the flower for several minutes without interruption, you begin to *become* the flower. You terminate the subject-object condition. There is no longer a "you" who is looking at a "flower"; your identity is no longer separate from that of the flower. You become the flower and effect Yoga with it. You and the flower are ONE and in this Oneness there is no "you" and there is no "flower." There only IS. Awareness emerges and separation dissolves. In your first few practice sessions with the flower you will probably be able to remain in this merged state for only a brief period. But even a few seconds will be a highly meaningful experience. Whenever this state of Oneness dissolves during your practice and the subject-object relationship returns ("I am a person looking at a flower"), make an intensive effort to merge again through total, unwavering concentration on the flower. Do not become tense, do not scold your mind for distracting you. Simply guide it back to the flower.

3. When approximately ten minutes have elapsed, slowly extend your legs and rest a few moments before rising. If, during the meditation period of ten minutes, your Lotus posture becomes uncomfortable, you can reverse the position of the legs. But do this in a way that will cause minimum distraction.

You need not confine this technique to the time and place of your meditation practice. It can be done in any situation where you find yourself sitting quietly—traveling, waiting in an office, resting during the day. Fix your gaze upon an object that is pleasing to your eyes and engage in the practice of close scrutiny and then mergence. Through this technique, your perception assumes a greater depth and the way you regard objects and people expands. It is as if you see another dimension of them and the manner in which all things are interwoven begins to be recognized. Separation is the illusion. All is One.

INCENSE

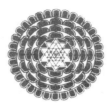

The third of the senses that we utilize for meditation is that of smell. An odor can have such a direct and profound effect that the mind becomes totally occupied with it and all other senses are rendered almost inoperative. This fact serves us well, because if you occupy the mind with an odor that requires its full attention, you nullify, to a great extent, the other senses that frequently prove distracting in meditation and you force the mind to block out other thoughts. It is as though a gentle emergency has been created with which the mind must become fully occupied.

The power of incense, in its various forms, has been recognized throughout the centuries and is used in a multitude of religious and secular contexts. The odor of burning incense in a place of worship immediately reminds the participant of the spiritual nature of that setting and assists him or her in transcending the ego in preparation for communing with the object of worship. Frequently incense impacts with such force that it acts as the medium to transport one into another dimension of consciousness. Our use of incense is for the first purpose stated above: We want to develop one-pointed fixation of the consciousness in a way that will prevent thoughts from arising. Let us reiterate here that our ultimate objective is not to permanently suppress all thoughts in our everyday activities. Rather, it is to recognize that thoughts are necessary to assist us in performing what we perceive to be our duties in life. But thoughts are not a part of us, they are not our Reality. They arise from the ego-shadow and they have no power to affect our true nature. When we understand thoughts from this perspective, they can do us no harm. But when we act upon thoughts as if we were an ego, then thoughts rule our lives and do us great damage, for they prevent us from being what we truly Are. It is to grasp this fact that we work, in meditation, to transcend thoughts so that we may have contact with the Reality that lies beyond them. In this way we gain a direct understanding of the nature of thoughts, the mind, and the ego, and we render their weapons ineffective. Thoughts and emotions come and go incessantly, but our Reality never comes or goes. It is eternal.

1. Obtain a supply of any incense that is pleasing to you. Place the lighted incense as close to your mat as necessary in order to detect the scent with ease, without it becoming overpowering. If necessary, adjust the distance during meditation. Sit in a Lotus posture. Practice Observation of the Breath for approximately two minutes.

2. Lower your eyelids so that just a slit of light remains. During the next ten minutes, fix your attention on and become totally involved with the scent, as you were previously involved with the flower. Determine if it is heavy, light, strong, subtle, sweet, and so forth. Take your time in noting these various qualities. Allow the scent to permeate your being. Now, as with the flower, we want to merge with the scent of the incense to effect Yoga (integration and absorbtion). Find that point at which there is no longer a "you" who is aware of the scent and a scent making itself known to you (subject-object). You and the scent are One. There are no longer thoughts about the scent. There is only Awareness, without beginning. This moment is eternal. It is not a point in the past-present-future sequence, but has always been and will always be. This is Pure Consciousness without limitations.

3. When approximately ten minutes have elapsed, slowly extend your legs and rest a few moments before rising.

It should be noted here that the time directions, for example, three minutes, ten minutes, etc., are approximations. They indicate the approximate minimal time you should spend with the techniques in your initial stages of practice. You may extend the sessions to as long as is comfortable. In the beginning students are inclined to measure their practice in terms of how many minutes should be allotted. At this point, they regard meditation as something that is apart from the mainstream of their lives. But as serious practice is continued, the student comes to recognize that meditation is the most meaningful activity in which he can engage, and as this recognition intensifies, the time allotted to meditation automatically increases. It is not unusual for students to meditate for an hour and more. But in the beginning you need not be concerned about this. From the moment you dedicate yourself to serious meditation practice, you will be guided by your inner Guru at each stage. This is a certainty because that Guru has been waiting for you to contact him or her through meditation.

TOUCH

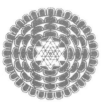

Using the tactile sense for meditation can be highly effective for those who are attracted to this type of contact. There is direct physical communication with the object of meditation. Those students who have difficulty with visualization and abstraction, or whose minds resist all efforts to become temporarily submissive, frequently find that touch meditation is the easiest technique to work with. Any small object that is pleasing and interesting, in terms of texture, shape, etc. may be used.

1. Place the object next to you. Sit in a Lotus posture and practice Observation of the Breath for approximately two minutes.

2. Take the object in your hands and close your eyes. During the next ten minutes fix your undivided attention on the object and become totally involved with it. Examine its qualities. Feel its weight, texture, form, temperature. Take your time with each quality and use all your fingers in the examination. Do not permit your attention to wander. As was the case with the candle, flower, and incense, we attempt to merge with the object we are contacting. If, without interruption, your mind and sense of touch have been totally involved with the object for several minutes, you should be able to *become* the object. Sink your consciousness into it. You are no longer making contact with the object, but the object and your consciousness have been integrated. You are not an individual self examining the qualities of an object. The mind and senses have been transcended and there is only Awareness. Attempt to maintain this condition of Oneness for the remainder of the session. If you lose the integration and the subject-object condition returns, merge again by total, unwavering one-pointed concentration on the object. Do not become discouraged if you are not immediately successful in achieving the integration. The practice is as important as the achievement because you are engaged in the process of disciplining and controlling the mind and senses, and this will result in noticeable benefits in all your daily activities. Remember that the mind and senses have run wild throughout your life and you must be patient in regaining control.

3. When approximately ten minutes have elapsed, open your eyes, slowly extend your legs, and rest a few moments before rising.

It is said by the *Gurus* that when the student understands the nature of contact, objects are no longer regarded as alien, separate entities, but are perceived only as an extension of the mind. The world is certainly within the mind that projects it. When you have recognized this fact, the world can hold no fear.

SURRENDER OF THE EGO

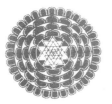

There are two paths in our meditation practice. The first is to discover the source of the mind, either through direct investigation (our next technique, "Where Am I?"), or by examining the mind's projections and merging with them. This latter method of mergence and transcendence is what we have been applying. The second path is a conscious surrender, a relinquishing of the ego-mind. The student requests, or petitions, that the ego be dissolved by offering it up as a type of sacrifice. This technique is particularly effective for those who are devotional, who may be attracted to prayer and worship, who have an insight into the nature of compassion, and who are inclined to be of assistance to others. The procedure is as follows:

Seated in a Lotus posture, practice Observation of the Breath for two minutes. Then visualize what for you is a representation of the Absolute. This symbol may be an image of a *Guru*, Jesus, Buddha, Krishna, a saint, a prophet, etc. Then, in your own words, petition the deity you are visualizing to guide you in understanding the unreality of your ego, to remove your illusions so that you may realize your Oneness with He who is being petitioned. You ask not that your desires be fulfilled, that you may become a better person, that you may reside in heaven, that your troubles in the world be resolved, but only that the ignorance preventing you from your recognition of Self be removed. You ask that the burden of the ego-shadow be taken from you. You repeat this request in your own words as many times as is comfortable during the meditation period. The visualization of the deity must be clear and steady. The mind must be totally occupied with it. If the visualization is weak, a replica—painting, picture, statue—may be placed where it can be easily seen and meditation can be practiced with the eyes fixed on it. But closing the eyes and *visualizing* the deity is preferable.

This technique initiates a purification process in which the mind impresses upon itself that it is a usurper, that it is posing as a monarch and attempting to rule a kingdom to which it has no rights. Continual reinforcement of this concept, by petitioning the deity to intervene, gradually loosens the tentacles of the ego; it continues to manifest, but with decreasing authority. The deity, when asked to do so, will in his own time and by his own methods dispell the illusion that the ego seeks to perpetuate. Once the deity is firmly fixed in your consciousness, you may surrender everything to him and dedicate all of your activities to him. "Not I, but Thou" becomes a guiding principle.

No special knowledge or preparation is necessary for this meditation. Simply visualize your representation of Self, the Absolute, and proceed as suggested above. It should be noted that the phrase "two paths," as it appears above, is used only relatively. In terms of the Absolute, there are no paths. There is only Self, Here and Now.

WHERE AM I?

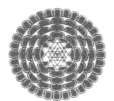

This technique involves direct investigation of the *source* of the mind. The question "Where Am I?" implies the seeking and finding of that place from where one's Reality emanates. People ask thousands of questions about things that are alien to their true natures, believing that the answers to these questions can eventually lead them to some extremely profound truth. But these answers only lead to more questions that require more answers that generate more questions, and so on without end. In Yoga there is only one question to be answered: "Where—or Who—Am I?" The answer to this question will put an end to all other questions.

During the time you allot to the meditation session, you silently ask yourself, "Where Am I?" This is a question that the computer, the mind, rejects as "illogical input." That is, it can respond immediately with the present location of your physical body and that's the end of it. It is not programmed to pursue the question further. This response of the body's physical location results from the mind being turned *outward*. It is seeking physical location in a physical world. But this is not the response we want. We are attempting to determine from where the "I" arises. What is its source? So we repeat the question, "Where Am I?" And the computer says, "I just told you. You are sitting here...." And you inform the mind that this is an unsatisfactory response, and you introduce the question again, and then again. You must be very attentive to what occurs, because the mind, sensing that there is some threat, will respond that there is no other answer to the question and will attempt to move on to other matters. Remember that it will do anything to avoid scrutiny. It is as slippery as an eel. It squirms, writhes, and wriggles out of any situation that threatens the omnipotent position it has assumed with the bravado of pure bluff. It cannot survive exposure. So we must persist. We must catch it and push it against the wall again and again and afford it no avenues of escape. Because it is flowing outward and seeing an external world, it is perfectly correct when it responds to the question by giving the location of your physical body. But what we are looking for is not in the body, nor in the world. We are seeking the source of the mind in a dimension that we may designate as "within." Therefore, we must continue to stun and confound it long enough to have it cease its outward flow and back up on itself. We maneuver it so that it has no alternative but to turn *inward*. This is accomplished by continuing to reintroduce the question "Where Am I?" Eventually the moment comes when the mind, exhausted by your persistence and unable to furnish the response that will enable it to free itself and resume its wildness, *will* back up on itself and turn inward. This moment represents a major development; from that point on, you can begin productive investigation.

Trace the source of the ego-mind as the great explorers traced the source of rivers. Find the lake, the Self, from where the river, the ego, originates. As the river flows into the lake or ocean and is absorbed therein, so does the mind flow into Self where it is dissolved. Once recognizing and merging with your source, the ego-mind and its thoughts can never again dominate you. Thereafter, whenever the mind "thinks," you know it can do so only as an aspect, a reflection of its source, Self, and you can never again be deluded by the dreams and fantasies of an ego.

How does one accomplish this tracing of the mind to its source? There is no roadmap. Nobody, however enlightened, can place you in your source. This is the adventure you must undertake by yourself. This is the true business of life. Someone can tell you to look at an object, but only you can do the seeing. Dive within and go into the depths, as a diver in search of treasure dives deep into the sea. Retrace your steps and go within the same way you have come out. Pemit nothing to divert you in your quest. Continue to inquire "Where Am I?" and do not stop until you have discovered *Who* is asking the question.

RICHARD HITTLEMAN

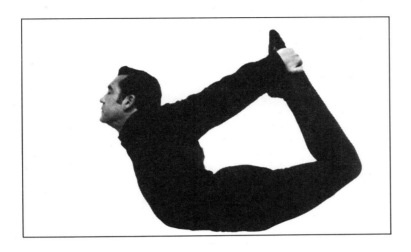

Born in New York City in 1927, Richard Hittleman began his study of Yoga at the age of nine, under the supervision of a Hindu employee of his parents. He continued the practice of Yoga while attending school and, after receiving his Masters Degree from Columbia University Teachers College, embarked upon a lengthy period of intensive study with Hindu *Gurus*. It was during these years that he developed the "Yoga For Health" system.

He founded his first school in Florida in 1957 and pioneered Yoga instruction via television with the "Yoga For Health" series, which premiered in Los Angeles in 1961. These programs, televised throughout the United States and in many foreign countries, have been instrumental in generating the significant growth of Yoga practice in the western world.

In addition to his television programs, Mr. Hittleman's books, lectures, and recordings have assisted in gaining national recognition of Yoga as a comprehensive system for holistic fitness and have drawn the attention of many medical and health authorities to its therapeutic value in various physi-cal and emotional problems.

Mr. Hittleman resides at the *Yoga Universal Ashram* in Northern California. He conducts special Yoga services and retreats and personally counsels serious adherants in the esoteric aspects of the Yoga doctrine.

For information regarding
Richard Hittleman's
Workshops and Retreats,
write to:

Yoga Universal
P. O. Box 66911
Scotts Valley, California 95066